Art Therapy with Veterans

of related interest

Music Therapy with Military Populations
Edited by Rebecca Vaudreuil
ISBN 978 1 787 75479 9
eISBN 978 1 787 75480 5

Moral Injury Reconciliation: A Practitioner's Guide for Treating Moral Injury, PTSD, Grief, and Military Sexual Trauma through Spiritual Formation Strategies
Dr Lewis Jeffery Lee
ISBN 978 1 785 92757 7
eISBN 978 1 784 50597 4

Art Therapy in Museums and Galleries
Edited by Ali Coles and Helen Jury
Foreword by Jordan Potash
ISBN 978 1 785 92411 8
eISBN 978 1 784 50775 6

Post-Traumatic Stress Disorder and Art Therapy
Amy Backos
ISBN 978 1 787 75204 7
eISBN 978 1 787 75205 4

ART THERAPY
WITH
VETERANS

EDITED BY
Rachel Mims

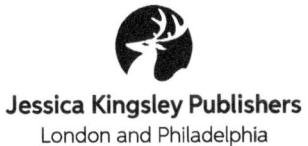

Jessica Kingsley Publishers
London and Philadelphia

First published in Great Britain in 2022 by Jessica Kingsley Publishers
An Hachette Company

1

Copyright © Jessica Kingsley Publishers 2022

A CIP catalogue record for this title is available from the
British Library and the Library of Congress

ISBN 978 1 787 75333 4
eISBN 978 1 787 75334 1

Printed and bound in the United States by Integrated Books International

Jessica Kingsley Publishers' policy is to use papers that are natural,
renewable and recyclable products and made from wood grown in
sustainable forests. The logging and manufacturing processes are expected
to conform to the environmental regulations of the country of origin.

Jessica Kingsley Publishers
Carmelite House
50 Victoria Embankment
London EC4Y 0DZ

www.jkp.com

Contents

Introduction

— RACHEL MIMS —

As I am a U.S. Army veteran and an art therapist, this book and the work it covers are very close to my heart. When I was in the military I was injured and had a very difficult recovery. Art is how I survived that recovery and was able to move on to other things after the military. This is not an uncommon story. Many veterans have utilized art to deal with physical and emotional pain. Many have used it to deal with the stresses of transitioning back to civilian life. For some, it gives a new purpose after leaving the military.

Packard (1980) wrote that the "power of art to transform human emotion was recognized as early as Plato's time" (p.11), but the healing potential of art making and/or the art object was not recognized until the 19th century. It was at this time that the connection between military service members, veterans, and artists began to be documented. In 1860, what was to eventually become the Artists Rifle Regiment in Britain was established (Lobban, 2017). By 1914 this regiment was an officer training corps that was comprised of multiple artistic professions. In 1916, a war artist's scheme was set up by the British Government to create propaganda, but by 1917 the war artists were instead recording and memorializing the war.

Adrian Hill, who served with the Artists Rifles and the Honorable Artillery Company (Lobban, 2017), became the first official war artist commissioned by the Imperial War Museum (Nicholls, 2020).

Hill continued to create art after World War I (Lobban, 2017). In 1938, he contracted tuberculosis and utilized art in his own recovery. As a result, he was invited to work with other war casualities. Hill is credited with coming up with the term "art therapy" (Lobban, 2017).

In the United States, art therapy with military veterans is documented as early as 1946 (Wix, 2000), at which time Mary Huntoon was appointed as the Director of Fine and Manual Arts at the Winter Veterans Administration Hospital. Huntoon served in this position until her retirement in 1958. Since this time, art therapy has been used to help this population heal from the wounds of war.

Although research on utilizing art therapy with military veterans has increased over the past several years, there is still a lot of information about working with this population that is unknown. This book aims to address an area that is currently lacking the literature. The chapters in this book address programs that are currently using art therapy in working with military veterans. The authors provide valuable information about how programs were implemented and how program participants have responded.

The book begins by addressing military sexual trauma (MST) and how group art therapy is being used to treat those who have experienced it. In this first chapter, I detail the history of sexual trauma within the U.S. military and review current literature on the topic. There is also an overview of a 12-week program I developed for use with survivors of MST.

Next, a museum-based art therapy program, Art for Warriors, is presented by Raquel Farrell-Kirk in Chapter 2. She details art therapy in museums, how the program was initially created and how it has evolved over time, and, using several case studies, she explores how it has impacted its participants. The chapter concludes with considerations for establishing new museum programs for veterans or service members.

The next chapter, Hand-Papermaking with Student Veterans, is presented by Meredith McMackin. She describes issues faced by student veterans and then details the use of hand-papermaking for therapeutic purposes. McMackin describes her doctoral research which included conducting a hand-papermaking workshop with student veterans. She then describes how the workshop impacted the participants.

Next, in Chapter 4, Jashley Boatwright discusses using an open studio art therapy approach with veterans. She details this approach and what it was like as a civilian intern and as a new art therapist to lead a veterans' group run by a non-profit organization. Boatwright then provides information on the experience of several of her group participants.

Erin Partridge then details her work with veterans in assisted living settings in Chapter 5. She discusses how to appropriately honor a veteran's service, how to deal with sudden disclosures, and how to recognize the veteran as whole person. She also provides information on dealing with the evolving memory of this population. Lastly, she discusses the role of the art therapist in this setting.

A relatively new topic to the literature, moral injury, is addressed by me in Chapter 6, which reviews literature on moral injury sources, impact, and assessment. I then discuss current treatments for moral injury and best practices, before moving on to look at the use of art therapy and creative methods in treating moral injury.

Next, in Chapter 7, Deborah Murphy discusses using a large-group art therapy format at a treatment facility for active-duty service members. She discusses the establishment of those programs as well as their ideology and application. She then details how the program functions during the weekly session. Lastly, she provides a wealth of information by giving sample directives that have been used in this program.

Art therapy in a military substance abuse rehabilitation clinic is detailed in Chapter 8, where Courtney Bennett and Kevin D'Augustine discuss their experience in this setting working with active-duty service members from all four branches. The chapter provides an extensive list of directives the authors have used and discusses how to facilitate these activities, as well as the typical outcomes the authors have observed.

For Chapter 9, the final chapter, several authors and I come together to address the issue of countertransference when working with military service members or veterans. I provide an overview of the topic and a short literature review. Then, Meredith McMackin, Gioia Chilton, Peter Buotte, and Kevin D'Augustine, each provide descriptions of their experiences working with this population and the countertransference they have experienced.

This book provides a wealth of knowledge about working with military service members and veterans in a wide range of settings. It is unique in that it addresses programs that currently exist and examines how they have been received by their participants. It is my hope that this book will provide inspiration for new programs working with military veterans so that more of them may experience the benefit of art therapy.

Chapter 1

Art Therapy Treatment for Military Sexual Trauma

— RACHEL MIMS —

The military has been aware of its sexual harassment problem since 1988 when the first U.S. Department of Defense (DoD) survey on sexual harassment found that during the previous 12 months, 64 percent of active-duty military women had experienced one or more unwelcome sexual behaviors. After the scandal surrounding the Navy Fliers' 35th Annual Tailhook Association's Convention in Las Vegas, Nevada, in 1991, DoD officials discussed conducting another study, but it did not take place until 1991 (Lancaster, 1999). Several more large-scale scandals occurred before the DoD changed its policies (U.S. DoD, 2004).

The DoD Sexual Assault Prevention and Response Office (SAPRO) was established in 2005. This office allowed for "a single point of accountability for sexual violence" (Turchik & Wilson, 2010, p.273). The SAPRO facilitates programs that give support and care to victims, and provides education, training, and prevention programming. This office set up the confidential reporting system for sexual assault that allows service members to file a report without notifying their command.

Even with the establishment of the SAPRO, sexual assault and sexual harassment are still prevalent in the military. In May of 2019, the DoD published the *Department of Defense Report on Sexual Assault in the Military: Fiscal Year 2018* (U.S. DoD, 2019). Results showed an increase in sexual assault of active-duty service women: 6.2 percent had experienced sexual assault in the year prior to being surveyed. "Using these rates, the Department estimates 20,500 Service members, representing about 13,000 women and 7500 men, experienced some kind of contact or penetrative sexual assault in 2018" (U.S. DoD, 2019, p.3). These numbers show that an estimated 30 percent of individuals do not make a report when assaulted.

Turchik and Wilson (2010) reviewed literature pertaining to the psychological effects of assault and found self-blame, shame, relationship problems, suicide ideation, and attempted suicide were common among victims of sexual assault. Additionally, victims of sexual assault were more likely to have increased levels of distress and physical health symptoms. Military sexual assault (MSA) was also linked to post-traumatic stress disorder (PTSD); Suris *et al.* (2004) found that women with a history of MSA were nine times more likely to have PTSD. Like MST, PTSD can greatly impact quality of life by increasing physical and emotional problems, family and social problems, and the chance of being homeless (Schnurr *et al.*, 2009). It is not just individuals who have experienced MST that are affected, but also those with whom the individuals interact: families, communities, and the nation as a whole are impacted.

This chapter presents an art therapy treatment program for women survivors of military sexual trauma. The following pages review relevant literature to support various elements of the program. Additionally, a session-by-session breakdown of the program is provided and includes pertinent information about how the author's previous clients have responded to the topics presented.

DEFINITION OF TERMS

The following terms are used throughout this chapter.

Military service member: An individual currently serving in any branch of the U.S. Armed Forces. The terms cadet and recruit are utilized to refer to military service members that have just recently begun their training.

Military sexual trauma: MST is defined as "psychological trauma, which in the judgment of a Veterans Affairs mental health professional, resulted from a physical assault of a sexual nature, battery of a sexual nature, or sexual harassment which occurred while the Veteran was serving on active duty or active duty for training" (U.S. Government Printing Office, 2006, p.261). According to the U.S. Department of Veterans Affairs (2014), MST includes any sexual activity where someone is involved against his or her will. This includes being pressured into sexual activities, or being unable to consent to sexual activities; for example, if intoxicated at the time. Unwanted sexual touching or grabbing, threatening and unwelcome sexual advances, and threatening, offensive remarks about your body or your sexual activities are listed as examples of MST (U.S. Department of Veterans Affairs, 2014).

Sexual assault: The DoD (2012) defines sexual assault as "a range of crimes, including rape, sexual assault, non-consensual sodomy, aggravated sexual contact, abusive sexual contact, and attempts to commit these offenses" (p.63).

Sexual harassment: In *Title 38 – Veterans' Benefits* of the U.S. Code, sexual harassment is defined as "repeated, unsolicited verbal or physical contact of sexual nature which is threatening in character" (U.S. Government Printing Office, 2006, p.262).

Veteran: An individual who has formerly served in the military.

LITERATURE REVIEW

The following section will review the literature that is relevant to the group art therapy program for the treatment of military sexual trauma (MST). First, military culture will be discussed with a focus on women in the military. Then, the consequences of MST will be detailed. Current treatments for MST are examined and the rationale for treating MST with group art therapy is provided. Finally, art therapy treatments for veterans and service members with PTSD are discussed.

Military culture and women in the military

Due to shared language, norms, and beliefs of military members and veterans, it has been said that the military constitutes a distinct culture. Although it is necessary for clinicians to be familiar with military culture when working with military members or veterans, there are unique aspects to consider when treating women with a history of MST. In this section, I will focus on the unique experience of women in the military.

Callahan (2009) wrote that the masculine warrior culture of the United States Air Force Academy (USAFA) required women to "unlearn almost two decades of socialization and adopt a persona that is counter to what they have been taught equates to success" (p.1159). Women in the military have conflicting role demands; they are expected to be attractive and feminine while upholding the masculine qualities that are equated with success in the military. Turchik and Wilson (2010) noted that a power differential between men and women results from the male-dominated structure of the military where men assume greater leadership roles. Women are an underrepresented minority and their historical exclusion from combat roles has prevented promotion to higher-ranking positions.

Sexual harassment in the military is so common that many women, like Callahan (2009), do not even realize it is occurring. Callahan stated that it was not until she was out of the military that she realized the "seemingly good-natured bantering about women and such topics as their bodies (including genitalia), their 'support roles' in the group, or their attendance at the USAFA as a means to earn a 'M.R.S.' degree" was a form of sexual harassment. Callahan was so accustomed to these behaviors that she did not acknowledge them as sexual harassment.

In the January 2019 *Industry Study Report*, Protect Our Defenders found that women reported that higher-ranking leaders and peers showed a lackadaisical and jovial attitude toward the topic of sexual assault and sexual harassment which facilitated trainings with crude jokes and laughter. This behavior, along with reports of other service women who shared their assault with supervisors and were not believed or retaliated against, demonstrates that assault and sexual violence are not taken seriously. One interviewee stated: "I had no idea where to turn, or who I could trust for support" (Protect Our Defenders, 2019, p.15).

Wanting to forget the event and move on, and not wanting more people to know about their assault are two of the reasons women give for not reporting (U.S. DoD, 2019). Other cited reasons for not reporting include fear of professional or social retaliation, not thinking it was serious enough to report, fearing that no action would be taken, difficulty accessing disclosure recipients, lack of desirable disclosure recipients, fear for personal safety, concern about embarrassing the military, and distress or shame (Dardis *et al.* 2018; U.S. DoD, 2020). These fears are not unfounded. In 2012, the DoD reported that of those who did file a report, 31 percent experienced social retaliation, and 26 percent experienced a combination of social retaliation, professional retaliation, punishment and/or administrative action.

MST and the U.S. Department of Veterans Affairs (VA)

The U.S. Department of Veterans Affairs (2014) began developing programs to screen and treat MST in 1992 and have since been training staff on MST-related issues and conducing outreach to veterans about available services. Currently, all veterans seen at the VA are screened for MST. All treatment for physical or mental health issues related to MST is free, unlike treatment for other ailments, which must be service-connected (having a VA disability rating) (U.S. Department of Veterans Affairs, 2014). Each VA healthcare facility has an MST coordinator who helps veterans access care. Every VA medical center and many VA community-based outpatient clinics offer MST-related outpatient services. Services offered include group and individual therapy, psychological assessment and evaluation, and medical evaluation and treatment.

Therapy is also available via the VA's community-based Vet Centers. Additionally, the VA offers MST-related mental health inpatient and residential treatment (U.S. Department of Veterans Affairs, 2019a).

What are the consequences of MST?

Unlike civilian sexual assault, MST typically occurs in the workplace environment. Therefore, MST victims are likely to have to see their perpetrator in both their workplace and their living quarters. Because perpetrators are often in the victim's chain of command, the victim's career may be interrupted if the person responsible for their evaluations and promotions is the attacker or a friend of the attacker. This can also result in not being granted access to care after MST. Often an MST victim must choose to have frequent contact with their perpetrator or sacrifice their career (U.S. Department of Veterans Affairs, 2004).

In a study that examined the universal screening program for MST used by the VA, Kimerling *et al.* (2007) found that MST was associated with two to three times greater risk of a mental health diagnosis. PTSD had the strongest association with MST. Several medical conditions were associated with MST: liver disease and chronic pulmonary disease were associated for both men and women, and women were more likely to be affected by hypothyroidism, obesity, and weight loss. Similarly, Middleton and Craig (2012) examined PTSD among female veterans and found MST and PTSD were strongly associated, and physical health was affected in those with PTSD.

Monteith *et al.* (2016) investigated the connection between perceptions of institutional betrayal and symptoms of PTSD, suicidal ideation and attempt, and depression after MST. Over 95 percent of the study participants reported experiencing institutional betrayal with MST, and this was significantly associated with symptoms of PTSD and depression as well as attempting suicide after MST (Monteith *et al.*, 2016).

Loss of identity is another characteristic unique to MST. Northcut and Kienow (2014) stated that becoming a military service member contributes greatly to how an individual views him/herself. Military culture creates a "sense of being protected and cared for by those in higher ranking positions" (Northcut & Kienow, 2014, p.249). The need to protect the collective often results in the group acting to preserve the status quo, which can result in re-traumatization as an MST survivor attempts to seek help. Monteith *et al.* (2016) reported "the institutional response after MST appears to be important because many Veterans indicated that they encountered difficulty reporting such experiences and no longer felt like a valued member of the military intuition after MST" (p.751).

MST treatment

A thorough review of several databases found that most articles that address MST treatment do so from the perspective of treating associated PTSD. The following section looks at treatments specific to MST.

WARRIOR RENEW

The Warrior Renew program (previously named "Renew") was developed as a 12-week, five-day intensive outpatient program to treat MST; an optional supportive housing program was available for homeless women veterans (Katz, 2016). Additional activities such as yoga, art, self-defense, health education, recreational outings, case management, and substance abuse groups were also available. Many researchers have studied Warrior Renew and found positive results. Katz *et al.* (2014) found significant reduction in negative symptoms, an increase in self-esteem and optimism, and higher life satisfaction. Katz *et al.* (2015) found that symptom reduction sustained 12-months from baseline, and self-esteem and quality of life increased over time. Katz (2016 p.367) found "significant decreases in perceived fearful and submissive insecure attachment, and significant increases in secure attachment."

TAKING CHARGE

Taking Charge consists of three-hour group sessions once a week for 12 weeks; in the pilot study the groups consisted of one hour each of psychotherapy, physical self-defense training, and group debriefing (David, Simpson & Cotton, 2006). Data from the outcome measures showed an increase in sense of personal safety, confidence in self-defense skills, confidence in ability to be assertive and set boundaries, ability to discern risky situations, and willingness to participate in community activities. Decreases were found for the following: obsessive fear and worry about assault, depression, and PTSD hyperarousal and avoidance symptoms (David *et al.*, 2006)

STAIR NARRATIVE THERAPY

According to Cloitre and Schmidt (2015), Skills Training in Affective and Interpersonal Regulation (STAIR) Narrative Therapy is an evidence-based treatment that has been found to be beneficial for individuals with PTSD from any type of trauma. Sessions 1–8 of STAIR Narrative Therapy focus on emotion regulation and social/interpersonal skills. Sessions 9–16 continue focus on skills training but also introduce the narration of traumatic experiences (Cloitre & Schmidt, 2015). STAIR with and without narrative therapy has been found to result in a clinically meaningful change in PTSD symptoms (Cloitre, Jackson & Schmidt, 2016). STAIR is also being used to treat MST via telemental health delivery (Weiss *et al.*, 2018). Results found that depression and PTSD symptoms were significantly reduced and emotional regulation skills were significantly improved.

COGNITIVE PROCESSING THERAPY (CPT)

"CPT is an evidence-based treatment for reducing PTSD symptoms related to various traumatic events" (Voelkel *et al.*, 2015, p.174). Researchers are examining CPT's usefulness in treating MST. Holliday *et al.* (2015) found using CPT to treat MST resulted in self-reports of significantly higher physical functioning. Suris *et al.* (2013) found a reduction self-reported PTSD symptoms. Although results are promising, more research is needed to determine if CPT is an effective treatment for MST.

Although there are some treatments specific to MST, there is an overall lack of literature on the topic. Middleton and Craig (2012) concluded that "Military Sexual Trauma and its relation to PTSD among female veterans is the most heavily researched topic" (p.248). Because of the strong tie between MST and PTSD, it is pertinent that anyone treating MST be familiar with PTSD treatment as well.

ART THERAPY TREATMENT FOR VETERANS WITH PTSD

Due to combat being a group experience, which typically results in traumatic experiences in a group context, group treatment of combat-related PTSD can be particularly useful. Group treatment provides empathy from other survivors, cohesion, and a safe environment for the sharing of traumatic material (Collie *et al.*, 2006; Smith, 2016). After working with Vietnam veterans with PTSD for over a decade, Rozynko and Dondershine (1991) also recommended group treatment of combat-related PTSD because it develops of a sense of belonging among members and provides a protective environment for the release of emotions. Ready *et al.* (2012) found that group treatment may be beneficial because of the commonly shared war-based knowledge that may not be possessed by a therapist who has not had first-hand experience with war. Additionally, group members may be more willing to accept the feedback of other combat veterans than that of a therapist without combat experience.

Group art therapy has the potential to aid those suffering from military-related trauma. Difficulty experiencing and expressing emotions is a common occurrence among those with a history of trauma. Art therapy offers the opportunity for non-verbal expression, which may aid in the accessing and processing of traumatic memories (Johnson, 2000). Collie *et al.* (2006) stated that art making is vital for the establishment of a trauma narrative because it allows for containment of traumatic material within an object or image, which promotes a sense of control and self-efficacy. Smith (2016) examined literature about the therapeutic mechanisms of art therapy for veterans with PTSD. A thematic analysis of 11 papers found that the group process provides for healing in ways that individual therapy does not, art therapy allows for the externalization of images, non-verbal expression via art facilitates verbal expression, creating art can assist in the integration of memories, and art making is pleasurable and results in a sense of mastery.

Until recently, most articles documenting art therapy treatment of veterans with PTSD were case studies (Avrahami, 2008; Berkowitz, 1990; Malchiodi, 2012). Lobban and Murphy (2018) found that a short-term group art therapy experience helped veterans with PTSD to overcome experiential avoidance. Walker *et al.* (2017) reported that art therapy provided a means of discussing "unseen wounds and struggles by referring to an object" (p.9). They also stated that group art therapy allowed participants to provide positive feedback to peers experiencing similar situations.

Jones *et al.* (2018) reported on the use of art therapy with military service members at the National Intrepid Center of Excellence (NICoE) and the Intrepid Spirit One (a satellite center of NICoE). The goals of the groups are "reducing isolation, building relationships, and increasing communication through the shared process of creating and talking about their artwork together" (Jones *et al.*, 2018, p.80). The authors reported that art therapy has helped their participants take a deeper look at what underlies their symptoms. Participants in these programs have reported that art therapy helped them find hope, experience positive emotions, and gain control over symptoms and experiences. In looking at survey responses from patients in these two programs, Kaimal *et al.* (2019) found that art therapy resulted in "positive changes in sense of self, interest in activities, anger, feeling depressed, ability to experience positive emotions, and feelings of guilt" (p.32). They also found that short-term art therapy resulted in improved aspects of identity and self-expression, while long-term art therapy was needed to address deeper issues.

Summary of the literature review

Literature relevant to the study of MST was reviewed, starting with military culture and women in the military. The consequences of MST were identified; they include a greater risk of a mental health diagnosis, increased chances of several medical conditions (Kimerling *et al.*, 2007), possible negative career impact, loss of identity and potential re-traumatization due to institutional betrayal (Monteith *et al.*, 2006; Northcut & Kineow, 2014). Next, current treatments for MST were discussed and a rationale for group art therapy treatment of MST was provided. Finally, art therapy treatment for veterans and service members with PTSD was detailed.

AN ART THERAPY GROUP TREATMENT FOR MST

The program described below is modeled on the Courage Group workbook written by Foley (n.d) to aid therapists conducting outpatient sexual trauma groups. The workbook includes suggested topics and activities for a 12-week group. The group art therapy treatment for MST also includes some topics which are typically addressed when treating PTSD with cognitive processing therapy (Resick, Monson & Chard, 2017). The goal of the program is to provide an MST treatment that addresses both verbal and non-verbal aspects of trauma in order to decrease symptoms that result from the MST, and therefore improve quality of life for participants.

Setting and participants

The program was delivered in a non-profit organization that provides counseling and social services for veterans and their families. Potential participants were identified by clinical staff and referred to the author; all participants were female veterans who had experienced MST. As suggested by Foley (n.d.), group sessions were conducted in one of the organization's group rooms that could accommodate the group size and contained a chalkboard, a dry erase board, or an easel with butcher paper. A session-by-session outline of the program is provided below with notes from the author.

Description of the procedures

The group art therapy treatment for MST follows a psychoeducational approach when discussing the weekly topics to facilitate group learning. A humanistic approach is utilized during art activities and trauma presentations to allow for an individual focus. The author identified short-term goals of building group cohesion and increasing knowledge of MST. Mid-term and long-term goals were to increase ability to identify emotions, improve relationships, enable the telling of the trauma story, and increase quality of life via reduction of trauma symptoms.

PRE-GROUP ASSESSMENTS

Prior to starting group, participants were screened by the author. A variety of assessments were completed to gather baseline data on clients. The Quick Inventory of Depressive Symptomology Report (QIDS-SR 16) and the Patient Health Questionnaire (PHQ-9) were utilized to assess symptoms of depression. Anxiety was measured via the Generalized Anxiety Disorder 7-item scale (GAD-7). Lastly, PTSD symptoms were measured via the PTSD Checklist for *DSM 5* (PCL-5) (American Psychiatric Association, 2013) past month version.

WEEK 1

As suggested by Foley (n.d.), during this session group rules are discussed and the group is guided in developing their own goals to reflect what they desire to gain from participating in the group. An overview of the program is given and participants then create "safe place" drawings, which represent a place where they feel safe. Next, sexual trauma is defined, treatment of sexual trauma is discussed, and the group talks about the effects of sexual trauma utilizing the session outlines provided by Foley (n.d.) as a guide. Lastly, the participants play a game designed to help them remember each other's names.

During this initial session, many of the clients are nervous as this is the first time they have elected to participate in a group. Providing the group with an overview of the program allows for reassurance that they will not be required to share their trauma story. Defining sexual trauma is important as there can be a lot of confusion about what constitutes sexual harassment, sexual assault, rape, and trauma. Finally, going over the effects of sexual trauma helps clients to begin to realize how MST has impacted them and that they are not alone in experiencing these effects. For example, one participant stated: "I always pushed it aside because it wasn't rape, but now I am realizing that it did impact me."

WEEK 2

The goal of this session is for group members to develop an understanding of emotions, anxiety, and depression. Psychoeducation on emotions, and the coping skills discussion and activity are facilitated using Foley's (n.d.) anxiety and depression outlines. Emotions are discussed via the use of several dialectical behavioral therapy handouts: emotion regulation handouts 3, 4A, 9, 16, and 22 (Linehan, 2015). Capacchione's (2002) "self-inventory" exercise is used to guide participants in creating lists of what they have accomplished that brings them pride. As homework, clients examine a list of possible self-care activities and identify which ones are feasible and might also be enjoyable. This session is important because it allows participants to acknowledge the positive aspects of their lives and begin a beneficial self-care practice.

The self-inventory exercise asks participants to make four lists: my skills and talents, my areas of knowledge and expertise, my positive personality traits and qualities, and my most important achievements (Capacchione, 2002). This usually causes some slight anxiety as participants worry if they will be able to "come up with enough" for each list. After starting though, clients are generally able to identify at least two things for each list. When sharing their lists, they often learn from each other and realize they have even more that they could add to their lists. Some example skills and talents identified by clients are cooking, making people laugh, reading, and growing houseplants. Example areas of knowledge and expertise identified by clients include psychology, quality assurance auditor-inspector, and military. Uplifting, humble, cheerful, and helping others have been listed by clients as positive personality traits and qualities. In the final column, "my most important achievements," clients have identified the following: realizing and seeking proper help, holding a top-secret clearance in the military, being the first in their military job field to pass training, and getting an honorable discharge.

WEEK 3

This session concentrates on anger and utilizes Foley's (n.d.) session outline for anger. The art activity in week 3 asks participants to draw their anger. Figure 1.1 is a representation of anger created by a client in an MST treatment group. At the end of this session, clients are given an assignment to write a letter expressing their anger to their perpetrator, non-protecting parent, or the military, and to bring the letter to the next session.

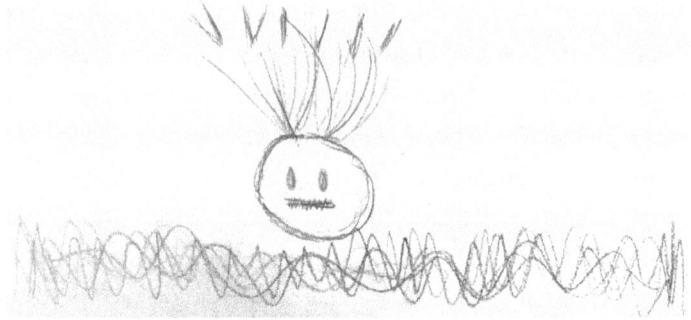

Figure 1.1: A client's representation of anger

WEEK 4

Self-esteem is the focus of week 4, and Foley's (n.d.) self-esteem outline is followed. Prior to starting on self-esteem, clients who are willing read the letters they wrote between sessions and the group discusses the letters. Next, clients create an image of themselves before the trauma and another one of themselves after the trauma. This particular exercise is hard for some clients because their experience with sexual trauma began at such a young age they are unable to remember themselves prior to the trauma. Figure 1.2 was drawn by a client who had no memory of life before trauma. On the top half of her paper, the before trauma image (not shown), she simply drew a small smiley face. The bottom half of her drawing (shown in Figure 1.2) shows her depiction of herself after the trauma.

During week 4, the group also creates a "Bill of Rights" where they complete the sentence "As a survivor of sexual trauma, I have the right to..." (Foley, n.d., p.35). The group completes this activity on a large sheet of paper using a variety of art materials. A Bill of Rights can be seen below in Figure 1.3. This activity helps group participants identify what they desire from life and realize that they have the right to go after it.

SHAME
ANGUISH
ANGER
FEAR
SELF RECRIMINATION
DEPRESSION
FLASHBACKS
GUILT

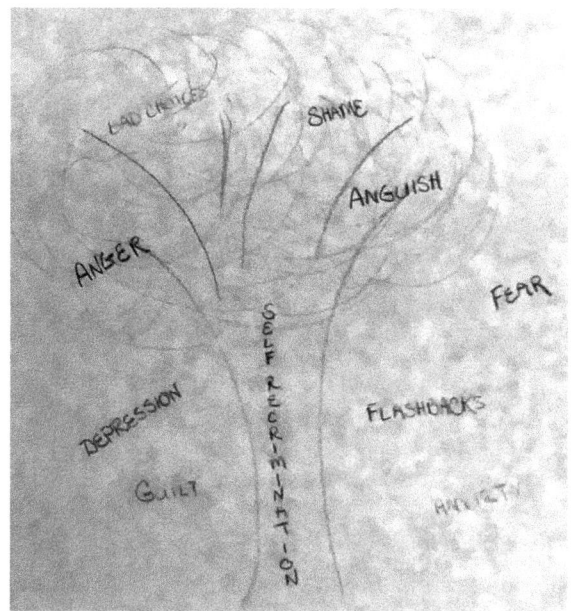

Figure 1.2: A client's before and after trauma drawings

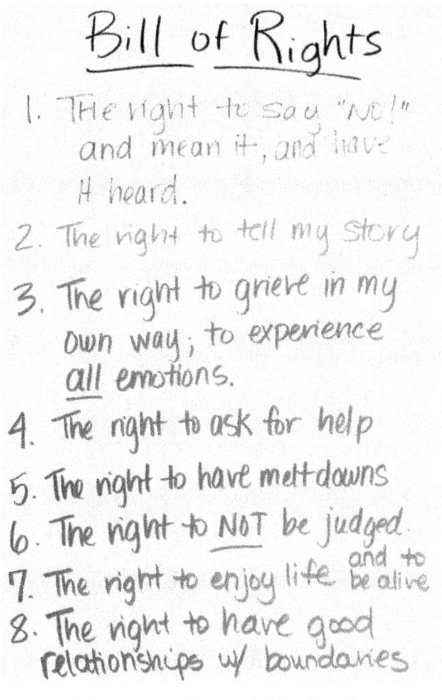

Bill of Rights
1. The right to say "NO!" and mean it, and have it heard.
2. The right to tell my story
3. The right to grieve in my own way; to experience all emotions.
4. The right to ask for help
5. The right to have meltdowns
6. The right to NOT be judged.
7. The right to enjoy life and to be alive
8. The right to have good relationships w/ boundaries

Figure 1.3: Group Bill of Rights

WEEK 5

During this session, Foley's (n.d.) relationships and intimacy outlines are followed. The art activity for this session is to create an image that represents a healthy relationship. Again, this activity may be difficult for some participants because of a long history of unhealthy relationships. A discussion of what they would like from relationships in the future may be beneficial.

WEEK 6

This session focuses on boundaries and assertiveness and utilizes Foley's (n.d.) outline. The activity during this session is a role play so that clients can practice responding to different situations in an assertive manner. The session concludes with a discussion that utilizes part of Foley's (n.d.) Breaking the Silence outline. Finally, any individuals who will be presenting their trauma experience during the next session are identified.

WEEK 7

This session allows group members to share previously undisclosed parts of their trauma experiences with each other. This is not required, and participants are reminded of this numerous times before this session occurs. As suggested in Foley's (n.d.) Breaking the Silence outline, each participant is asked to bring a photo of themselves from around the time of the abuse. Session length is long enough to allow two to four participants to share their experiences with each other. If the group comprises more individuals, or those who like to provide a lot of details, additional sessions may be required. The author suggests adjusting weeks 7–10 based on group size and desired content in order to accommodate additional sessions for sharing trauma experiences.

Anxiety over sharing part of one's trauma story is common and group members have reported that knowing they were going to talk about their trauma resulted in increased symptoms between sessions. This session can, however, be very powerful. One client brought in a photo of herself as a teen; she stated that this was taken around the time of abuse from a particular perpetrator. The client stated that this was the only photo from when she was young. After telling the group about her experience around this time, she asked if she could destroy the photo. She was told she could do whatever she wanted with her photo and she decided to tear it up into small pieces. Afterwards, she expressed relief at having it out of her life.

WEEK 8

During this session, psychoeducation on trust is provided using the trust issues module from *Cognitive Processing Therapy for PTSD: A Comprehensive Manual* (a CPT workbook) by Resick *et al.* (2017). A discussion of Resick *et al.*'s (2017) concept of stuck points takes place and clients are asked to identify any trust-related stuck points they may have. During this session, one client stated: "I'm ready to break down the wall of flat affect I have been using to protect myself."

WEEK 9

This session begins with reviewing trust-related beliefs as discussed during the previous session. Clients complete a romantic relationship-focused trust star based on the trust star worksheet developed by Resick *et al.* (2017). Clients are asked to identify the many different types of trust they need to have in their romantic partner. They are then asked which types of trust are most important. Next, they rate someone they know on these trust continuums. Following the trust star exercise, a discussion of how trauma impacts safety-related beliefs takes place using the safety issues module developed by Resick *et al.* (2017).

WEEK 10

This session focuses on how trauma impacts esteem, intimacy, and power and control-related beliefs and uses Resick *et al.*'s (2017) applicable modules as outlines. After this discussion, clients are asked to identify three important things that PTSD has taught them. Some answers given by clients are: "I'm broken, but I'm still fighting," "I'm stronger than I thought I was," "I have abilities I never knew I had," and "I have learned more than I thought I could."

WEEKS 11 AND 12

The final two sessions are devoted to creating mixed-media masks to represent the clients' true selves. In the final session, the group is given a chance to discuss the meaning of their masks and reflect on their experiences with the group. One client chose to represent how she felt her MST experience had robbed her of her senses; she was not heard or seen by others and even felt that thinking was difficult. Figure 1.4 shows how she represented this on the inside of her mask. Another client stated that she tried to hide her despair but knew that it did show through so she added it to her mask. She also used the mask to show "I'm cracking and I am broke and trying to put my life back together." This mask can be seen in Figure 1.5.

Prior to leaving, group members complete the same assessments they completed for the pre-assessment. This allows the clinician to have quantitative data showing any change in symptoms that occurred while participating in the group. Although no research studies have been completed, the author has seen that participation in this group can result in a dramatic improvement for some individuals.

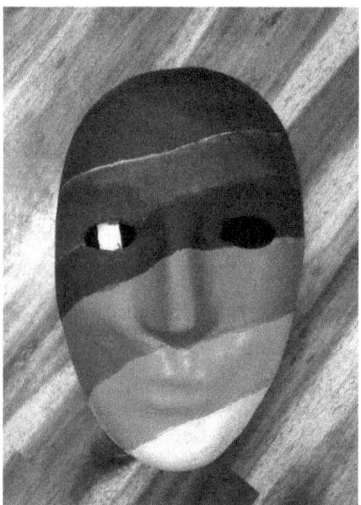

Figure 1.4: Client mask representing how MST robbed her of her senses

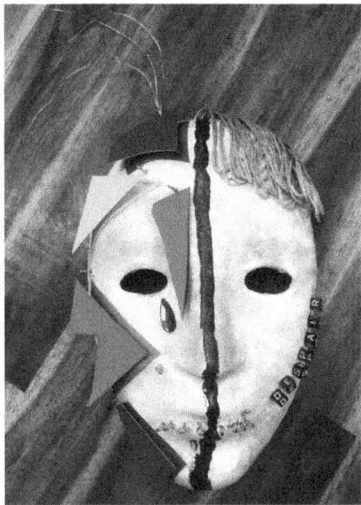

Figure 1.5: Client mask showing her despair

CONCLUSION

Because of the large number of individuals who are subjected to MST each year, an effective treatment is needed. Because art making enables individuals to view their traumatic experiences in a new way, art therapy can be an effective treatment for MST. This chapter reviewed literature to support the use of art therapy in a group format to treat MST. Lastly, the author detailed a 12-week group art therapy treatment for MST modeled after Foley's (n.d.) Courage Group workbook and some modules from cognitive processing therapy (Resick *et al.*, 2017). There are currently no research studies using this treatment, but improvement in patient quality of life has been observed by the author.

Chapter 2

Art for Warriors: A Museum-Based Art Therapy Program for Veterans

— RAQUEL FARRELL-KIRK —

INTRODUCTION
Veterans and art therapy

In a Pew Research Center survey, 27 percent of veterans, and 44 percent of those who served between 2001 and 2011, reported difficulty reintegrating into civilian life (Morin, 2011). In the 2019 Annual Member Survey of the Iraq and Afghanistan Veterans Association (IAVA), 78 percent of respondents reported at least some difficulty transitioning out of the military (IAVA, 2019). These concerns are particularly alarming in light of recent research demonstrating a link between veteran suicide and difficulty transitioning after military service (Reger, Smolensky & Skopp, 2015). Reintegration difficulties can center on strained relationships with loved ones as veterans struggle to regain their footing among families and communities where roles have changed or where others expect the veteran to return unchanged (Duttweiler, 2020). These same loved ones and community members often do not understand military culture and therefore fail to fully appreciate the extent to which leaving it can create anxiety and a loss of purpose (Coll & Weiss, 2013; Kopytin & Lebedev, 2013). When it comes to their communities at large, some veterans deem civilians "uninformed and in denial" (DeLucia, 2016, p.5) and suggest that collective trauma contributes to society's difficulty supporting veterans. These combined challenges have dire consequences, with the Department of Veteran's Affairs reporting that the suicide rate for veterans in 2017 was one and a half times that of the general adult population (U.S. Department of Veterans Affairs, 2019b).

In addition, it is estimated that almost 30 percent of those veterans who serve in combat may develop post-traumatic stress disorder (PTSD). Relatedly, 35 percent of Iraq war veterans sought mental healthcare within the first year of their return (Collie *et al.*, 2006). Stigma remains a barrier for veterans, with as many as 50 percent of recent veterans who report significant symptoms not seeking out treatment (Kulesza, Pedersen & Marshall, 2015). A small percentage of Vietnam veterans were still suffering from PTSD more than a decade after that conflict ended (Dohrenwend *et al.*, 2006), and prevalence of PTSD remains many times higher among deployed versus non-deployed veterans, even after ten years (Mandic-Gajic & Spiric, 2016). There may also be delayed recognition by the veteran and their loved ones that behaviors exhibited are indicative of PTSD and suggest a need for treatment (Smith, 2016). These statistics suggest long-lasting and significant challenges with trauma may impact the veteran population at a greater rate than the 3.5 percent PTSD prevalence rate reported for the general adult population (American Psychiatric Association, 2017). For those who do face PTSD and related symptoms, it is important that the nation works to provide effective and accessible care (Collie *et al.*, 2006)—not only to alleviate the human suffering toll PTSD extracts from veterans and their loved ones, but also because it is estimated that PTSD costs the nation's economy as much as $10,000 a year per veteran (Eibner, 2008).

Veterans dealing with PTSD may experience emotional numbing. PTSD-related emotional numbing doesn't just protect from difficult feelings, it robs one of pleasurable emotions as well. It can include disinterest, disconnection, and withdrawal from activities and interpersonal interactions (Center for Substance Abuse Treatment, 2014; Smith, Robinson & Segal, 2019).

A review of the literature on the efficacy of art therapy suggests it targets many of the symptoms and struggles impacting returning veterans that are described above. Art making can enhance mood, reduce anxiety, and relieve stress. Art products can symbolically contain stressors, promoting distance between oneself and one's problems as a step towards mastering them (Abbott, Shanahan & Neufeld, 2013; Bell & Robbins, 2007; Curl, 2008; Drake, Coleman & Winner, 2011; Kaimal, Ray & Muniz, 2016; Kopytin & Lebedev, 2013; Sandmire et al., 2012). Externalizing one's problem or difficult emotional material by creating art about it can provide safety, distance, choice on how to engage with or not engage with the problem, and a new perspective on the problem itself (Kopytin & Lebedev, 2013; Lobban, 2016). As one participant stated, prior to making art he had "carried his feelings and memories inside of him, but that now he was able to show this image to people and talk about it" (Canto et al., 2015, p.160). Trauma often results in memories that are encoded as fragmentary sensory content, lacking in verbal explanations or context. Art therapy, with its focus on imagery and direct engagement of the senses, may be uniquely equipped to access this largely non-verbal information and promote the integration of trauma memories (Lobban, 2016).

Group art making can build connections, decrease isolation, and help overcome resistance to art making (Haessler, as cited in Kopytin & Lebedev, 2013; Ramirez, 2016). In the case of veterans who are working through trauma, it is possible that group art therapy can provide "a container for the feelings of the group, being large enough to withstand the combined experiences of trauma for each member" (Smith, 2016, p.68). In addition, the cohesion found in a consistent art therapy group might mirror the group-based experience of military members who are used to functioning within units and battalions and can help them learn to re-establish trusting relationships. Creating art and discussing it in a group also normalizes participants' struggles (Lobban, 2016; Palmer et al., 2017). Art therapy's direct engagement with the pleasurable sensations and activities of art making may mitigate the emotional stress of exploring traumatic material and provide relaxation.

This aligns with research suggesting that treatment for emotional numbing should include pleasurable activities (Collie *et al.*, 2006; Kashdan, Elhai & Frueh, 2006; Mandic-Gajic & Spiric, 2016).

Awareness of the impact of art and art therapy on veterans is growing, as evidenced by features in mainstream media outlets such as National Geographic, TED talks, and the Huffington Post, the emergence of institutions like the National Veterans Art Museum, and the creation and growth of programs by the National Endowment for the Arts (NEA) (McGonigal, 2016; NEA, n.d.; Walker, 2015). VA physicians are finding art therapy valuable, as are veterans (McElveen, 2007). Studies about veterans receiving art therapy in the UK, and individual case studies, suggest that art therapy has therapeutic benefits for this population. National arts organizations have highlighted art and creative arts therapies as effective supports and beneficial resources for military members and their families in a wide range of settings (Klein, 2015; Levy *et al.*, 2018). This includes the National Initiative for Arts and Health in the Military's (NIAHM) observation that "providing service members and veterans with opportunities to express themselves and share their stories can help them cope with the most common symptoms of today's conflicts: post-traumatic stress (PTS), traumatic brain injury (TBI), and major depression" (NIAHM, 2013, p.19).

Klein (2015) notes that this growing attention led to a 2012 military roundtable regarding art and art therapy for veterans which resulted in a statement that:

> Unlike exposure-based therapies, when using the arts, individuals can experience and/or express their thoughts and feelings without necessarily having to talk about or directly confront the trauma... Participating in pleasurable activities also addresses emotional numbing, another feature of PTS—a lack of interest in activities, detachment from others, and a restricted range of emotional expressiveness. (NIAHM, 2013, p.21)

The existence of the National Veterans Art Museum in Chicago (NVAM), which exhibits artwork from veterans with PTSD, also speaks to this increasing awareness of the important role of art in the lives of veterans (Sloan, 2013).

Art therapy in museums

Museums have a long history of attempts to engage and support their communities, and a recently sharpened focus on supporting the diverse needs of their communities via accessibility and support of community healthcare issues (American Alliance of Museums, 2018; Merendino & Clark, 2010; Silverman, 2010). In fact, Montreal's Museum of Fine Arts recently made headlines when it hired a full-time art therapist as part of a program of "social prescriptions" where doctors might prescribe museum visits to patients (Vartanian, 2019). The American Alliance of Museums (2018) prioritizes "service to the public" as one of the top functions of the museum and states that "it is not enough anymore to appeal to a small, homogeneous audience. There is an expectation that any museum serves some broader slice of society" (p.20).

Gail Anderson, museum historian likens this to "dismantling the museum as an ivory tower" and re-imagining it as "a more socially responsive cultural institution" (Anderson, 2004, p.1). Similarly, Stephen Weil's 1999 article title summarizes this trend as moving "from being about something to being for somebody." Other authors highlight the increased focus being placed on this emerging role by museum professionals (Chatterjee & Noble, 2016).

This shift is borne out in both training programs producing new museum professionals and in the programming of current museums. Museum studies programs may now include visitor-centered frameworks and specifically mention social consciousness and social justice terminology in their training goals (Florida State University, 2019). Existing museum professionals are increasingly helping their institutions to address public health and social justice concerns, design programming with special populations in mind, and often view these programs as important tools in the quest to remain accessible and relevant (American Alliance of Museums, 2018; Naudziunas, 2013). Examples of the growth of specialized museum programming include the "Meet me at

MOMA" program at New York's Museum of Modern Art (n.d.) and "Met Escapes" at the Metropolitan Museum of Art (2019), both created specifically for those living with dementia and their caregivers. Sloan (2013) enumerates many more examples of specialized programming in museums ranging from New York to Australia and incorporating populations from children with autism to adults with developmental disabilities. Museums can use art therapy partnerships to support these efforts to increase access and reach under-served populations.

The British Art Therapy Association's (BAAT) Museum and Gallery Special Interest Group (2013), identifies specific roles for art therapists in museums. These include helping improve such factors as emotional engagement from visitors, access for those with mental health diagnoses and related issues, funding and educational offerings, and connections between sectors of our communities. From the point of view of the art therapist, art museums can be an impactful place to house art therapy programs (Ruehrwein, 2013). Placing art therapy within a museum highlights the central role of art in art therapy, and combats the stigma associated with seeking help (Patmali, 2017; Salom, 2011). Artwork in a museum's collection can be used to invite self-exploration and show that others have struggled with similar feelings, which suggests hope. Art therapy programming utilizes the otherwise unfulfilled potential of a museum's spaces, resources, and holdings to provide refuge, inspiration, and recovery (BAAT, 2013; Hamil, 2016; Melton, 2013; Patmali, 2017; Peacock, 2012; Rosenblatt, 2014; Salom, 2011).

This concept of the museum as a refuge is echoed in discussions of museum-based art therapy programs as inviting introspection and encouraging quiet contemplation of both artwork and personal meanings, and seems to be implied in reports that museums in New York saw a spike in attendance after the 9/11 attacks (Sloan, 2013). Silverman (2010) has explored and expanded on the potential roles of museums, and has noted that they help promote relaxation, invite introspection, and even encourage recollection. The provision of a "soothing atmosphere" has been cited as having a positive impact on veterans in art therapy and seems to be in line with most museum spaces with their open galleries, natural light, and orderly displays (Palmer *et al.*, 2017). The museum as inspiration echoes the art therapist's existing knowledge borne from facilitating group art therapy experiences where witnessing another's creative process and resultant product can lead to increased introspection and engagement in one's own art making (Parashak, 2013).

Museum-based art therapy programs promise additional benefits for veterans, cultural institutions, and communities. Veterans can gain awareness of museums as accessible, affordable options for recreation, socialization, and education, and can utilize museum resources to access art making, artwork, and art therapists. The museum setting can legitimize art making, decrease the stigma around services, decrease isolation and encourage dialogue between civilians and veterans. Connecting to a museum can serve as an important and sometimes first step in a larger effort to reconnect to a community and reintegrate into civilian life. The needs of veterans and communities, available resources and goals of cultural institutions, and benefits of art therapy combined to give rise to the Art for Warriors program.

PROGRAM OVERVIEW

Coral Springs Museum of Art first created the Art for Warriors program in 2015 as a multi-modal arts-based outreach program. In the program's first iteration, the program team did not include an art therapist, and activities ranged from spoken word and storytelling to dance. All sessions were held off site at veterans' organizations around the community. In 2016, the museum administration decided to reinvent it as a museum-based program, wanting to include the potential positive impact of the museum's physical spaces and changing art exhibitions in the program in order to further benefit participants. The museum's executive director and I had previously collaborated on an art exhibit at a different institution, highlighting the therapeutic benefit of art. Recalling this introduction to the formal field of art therapy, the executive director reached out to explore how a credentialed art therapist might enhance the program. The hope was that bringing an art therapist on board would help solidify the program's structure and goals, provide a theoretical base, and help with data collection and program evaluation. Thus, Art for Warriors became the museum's first art therapy program and is now one of three art therapy programs that operate at the museum each week. These programs are the only ones of their kind in South Florida and are part of just a handful of museum-based art therapy programs across the country.

The program was initially envisioned as a six-week-long closed group with a specific series of art directives planned for each of the six weeks. However, due to its popularity and efficacy, the museum sought and obtained continued funding and the program in its current version has been now been running for three consecutive years. The grant provides for a paid art therapist. Weekly sessions are held at the museum after hours (on Thursdays from 6:30pm to 8:30pm) in its spacious art studios, and all art materials are included. This two-hour time slot was chosen to ensure adequate time for both art making and discussion.

Once the initial six-week period passed and the program was renewed, the decision was made to focus on reaching as many veterans as possible and to remove as many barriers to attendance as possible. Active-duty and retired military members from any branch of the service and any conflict or era are welcome to attend. It is an open group where attendees are free to come and go from week to week and no formal pre-registration or commitment is required. This has helped promote the sense that the program, and the museum itself, is a reliable and consistent source of support. Groups are held year-round, only closing if holidays fall on our typical Thursday evening class schedule. This consistency has helped create a sense of safety and trust, which is integral to any therapeutic relationship but can be hard to develop in veterans who have been trained to keep their guard up.

Art for Warriors' overarching program goal is to provide relief from a range of stressors related to the participants' experience as veterans. The group serves as a supportive community that combats their isolation and provides stress relief through art making. It also introduces veterans to a variety of art media and techniques and their role in self-care and stress management. Since the museum sponsors and hosts the program, veterans' perceptions of museums and cultural institutions may also be transformed, allowing these institutions to be seen as affordable and accessible community resources.

PROGRAM DESCRIPTION AND PROCEDURES

Originally, the program had a prescribed art therapy directive each week. As the program continued beyond the original six-week time frame, and participants became more and more comfortable with the studio space, each other, and the art therapist, they began to take more and more ownership of their creative process and the group structure was altered. Members seemed to be settling into a new role: that of artist. Often, they would begin setting up their work area before any prompts or directives had been provided, and they seemed to take great pride in welcoming new members and giving them a tour of the supplies. The adoption of this new role is therapeutic in and of itself as it can be a welcome respite from being perceived, by self or others, as the one in need of help, or of being seen only as a one-dimensional version of themselves, only as a veteran.

Currently, a typical session begins with participants entering a few minutes before the starting time and socializing informally, often by either making coffee or helping themselves to the refreshments that are made available each week. There is a sign-in sheet that helps record attendees (average attendance is between five and seven) and if new attendees are present, initial paperwork such as consent forms are provided for them. Then participants gather at the tables and a brief check-in is completed, where each member is asked to rate their day or how they are feeling, on a scale from 0 to 10. Once housekeeping items such as these are complete, and participants have been welcomed and introductions made, a theme is introduced to help guide their art making. I often remind my group participants that though I may offer a theme, they are free to choose to alter it or stray from it in any way they like. This is an important acknowledgement of the fact that the client has a world outside the weekly visit to this group that the therapist is not privy to. Unlike a more intensive clinical setting where the client's week might be well known to the therapist, I do not know what each person's life holds for them outside our sessions. I am not part of a clinical team poring over intakes and comparing notes with other providers who are working with the same client. Therefore, I am not selecting an individualized art therapy directive based on in-depth knowledge of a client's needs. I am offering structure and guidance to allay anxieties related to unfamiliarity with art making, highlight widely applicable themes such as coping skills and self-care, and explore a range of accessible media and techniques.

The bulk of the session is spent in active art making. During each session, the art therapist circulates throughout the entire group to check on participants, offer technical assistance, explore themes and emotions that might be emerging in their artwork, and help establish and maintain rapport. Some evenings the mood of the group is light and social with lots of banter and conversation during art making; other times attendees work in quiet concentration on more emotionally charged pieces. For example, recently we had a talkative and social group where members shared favorite holiday traditions and memories. Just a week or two prior, the museum had a photojournalism exhibit based on the Marjory Stoneman Douglas High School shooting and half of the group was spent discussing trauma, gun violence, and self-care. Additionally, at the close of each session, participants often verbally process their artwork with the group. Participants are also expected to actively participate in cleaning up their work areas. The group session typically ends with a relaxation exercise such as a brief meditation or deep breathing techniques.

PROGRAM IMPACT

Generally, members' feedback about the group has been overwhelmingly positive, describing it in our written surveys and questionnaires as "amazing, relaxing, and educational" with comments such as "We need this," "This is my time for myself each week," and "This is the only time I am not thinking about all the other things on my mind." It should be noted, however, that positive bias is inherent in questionnaire formats (Palmer *et al.*, 2017). Evaluative comments, while anonymous, are collected by the art therapist. Efforts to find more objective and quantifiable ways to measure the program's impact are ongoing. The individual summaries and reflections shared below also provide helpful information on the impact of the program.

BRIAN (PSEUDONYM)

Brian is a Vietnam veteran who has attended the group with his wife since its inception in its current form. Spouses are welcome to attend our programs and his wife Kay has become a vital member of the group as well. They are both sociable and easy to engage in art making. Brian demonstrates artistic skill and talent and has a history of drawing and painting both for himself and his own enjoyment as well as for others. He is softly spoken but shares his wife's sense of humor. Brian is reserved and though he always participates in art making one could misinterpret it and assume that he is engaged in a superficial manner, socializing and creating artwork for relaxation. Though likely an error many would make, it would be wrong to assume that any trauma, sadness or other issues related to his service might long since have been resolved by previous treatment or the passage of decades. Brian gave important, though rare, glimpses that there was more to his relationship with the group than that. On one occasion, a funding organization invited one of our group members to film an interview about their participation in Art for Warriors that the organization would then play during a well-attended public event. Brian volunteered for the interview and shared about his service as a young man as well as about the impact of his weekly attendance at the group. He acknowledged in that interview that although service members may form wonderful bonds and see good things during their service, they often witness difficult things. As he put it, "The bad things, I think you have to spend about 50 years trying to get them out of your head." He added that some weeks, the art projects "get the guys talking and that's what helps a lot of the post problems that we have. It really helps. It's a good program." In preparation for this interview Brian had to gather mementos and old photographs from his time in service to share with the makers of the video. He and his wife took the opportunity to bring these items to the group one evening and he shared them with me in a private one-on-one conversation. The trust and intimacy of this sharing was extremely touching to me, especially as it was an invitation extended only to me. I learned a great deal from that exchange, and was reminded, in a very visceral way, of the staggering youth of many of these Vietnam veterans at the time of their deployment.

Brian often produced aesthetically pleasing artwork and participated in the two art exhibits we have held thus far for the program. For our first exhibit, he displayed his mask (Figure 2.1), a striking black and white portrayal that includes a tear, the image standing in stark contrast to his demeanor in group. Having the outlet to create this mask in a safe setting where he trusted that he was in control of how much he discussed or revealed allowed him to portray the tear and at least acknowledge his emotions in that way. Placing that tear on the mask, and hanging that mask in the exhibit, was quite a public display of emotion from such a quietly pleasant gentleman.

Brian's wife also participated in the exhibit, adding a three-dimensional piece I encouraged her to submit. We had completed a directive titled "Walk a Mile in My Shoes," where participants transformed shoes into works of art aimed at depicting something about themselves or their lives that others might not know, realize, or acknowledge. Kay transformed a tall, lace-up boot reminiscent of combat boots into a mountain being scaled by army men. She painted an expressive face on the back, and the climbing plastic army men on the front. She explained that the front of the shoe, with the army men scaling the mountain, represented the young men at the beginning of their service. In contrast, the expressive face on the back of the boot represented the men after their experiences (Figures 2.2 and 2.3).

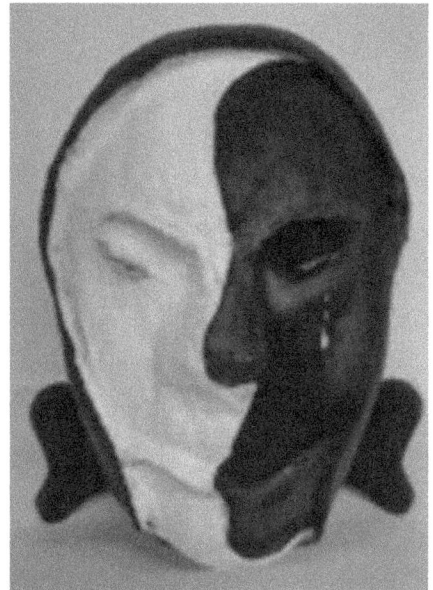

Figure 2.1: Brian's mask

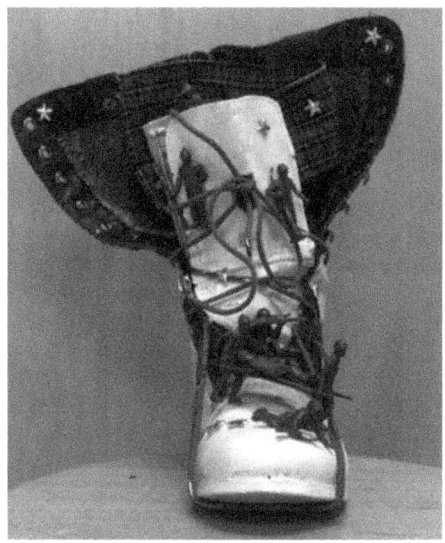

Figure 2.2: The front of Kay's boot

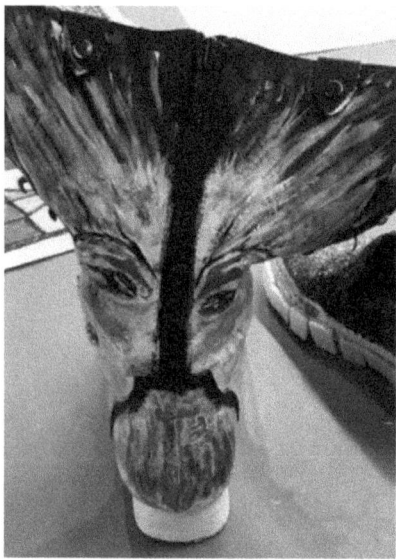

Figure 2.3: The back of Kay's boot

Attending as a couple provided Brian and his wife with a stress-free way to spend time together. While his military experience was something she may have struggled to relate to since they did not share or experience it as a married couple, the art therapy groups helped them develop their common interest in art and art making. They shared with the art therapist about family stressors and even significant losses of loved ones, so the group also served as a source of support.

BARBARA (PSEUDONYM)

Barbara began attending the program after finding the flyer at her local Veterans Affairs (VA treatment facility. An expressive personality and wonderful storyteller, she gave a charming account of how the flyer literally came to be stuck to her as she stood at the VA, seemingly to ensure that she found the program. She had long been a prolific artist and her comfort with art making and painting in particular made itself evident in her technically sophisticated and expressive paintings. She shared that she had been involved in clean-up efforts following 9/11 and that since that time her artwork had become monochromatic, symbolically mirroring the gray ash and metal she had been surrounded with and the internal darker emotional state she had entered. During her time with the group, however, what had begun as a gray and white painting of a female face was gradually transformed to include yellow rays of hope and vibrant red lips (Figure 2.4). She beamed as she observed with a smile that this was the first time she had painted in color.

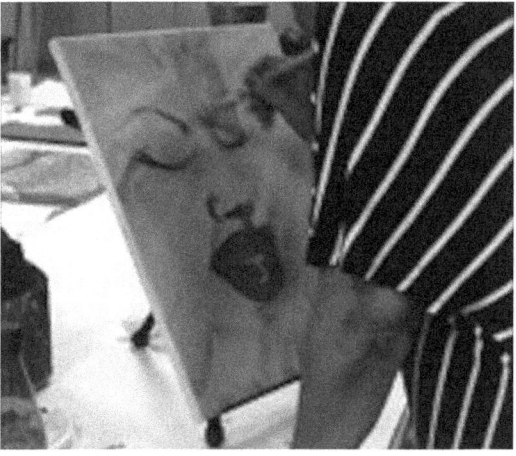

Figure 2.4: Barbara's painting

Over the course of the next several months to a year, Barbara participated in the group whenever she was in town, sharing her time between living with family members in South Florida and residing in her home outside the U.S. Eventually, she built on her success in the Art for Warriors program and ventured out to participate in other community-based endeavors, such as signing up to participate in a special training series for artist entrepreneurs. She reflected recently that the successful experience at Art for Warriors led her to approach new opportunities with the thought, "If I could do this [Art for Warriors], then I could do that." She continued doing one new thing at a time, repeating her mantra that each thing she accomplished was proof she could do the next thing, and in this manner, talked herself into participating in an art-making workshop for veterans conducted by a regionally known professional artist. In her words:

"From there I mean, there was such a scope, it was like a horizon that widened out...it snowballed." She is now pursuing art more formally and has enrolled in degree-seeking courses at a local college, managing general education requirements as well as the studio art classes that form the core of her degree.

ELLE (PSEUDONYM)

Elle joined the group recently and on her first evening was the only woman and the youngest veteran present. She was quiet and reserved in her discussion of artwork during the group but showed, via her smiles, that she enjoyed the banter that several of the group members had with each other. At the close of the group on her first evening she approached me to let me know that she had enjoyed the evening but would be unable to attend the following week unless she could bring her young daughter with her. She quickly assured me that the girl was quiet and well behaved and would be unobtrusive. I let her know that though I understood her co-nundrum, the group had tried an iteration that included younger children of veterans and had come to the conclusion that it was not compatible with the goals and design of the program. I told her I hoped she could join us again in the future but that it would have to be limited to evenings when she could attend without her child. She nodded politely, assured me she understood and then immediately burst into tears and ran from the room, declining to talk any further.

The museum's program coordinator and I both reached out to her via phone to follow up the next day. We were debating how to meet her obvious need for more support within the constraints of our program. As luck would have it, she let us know that due to some visitation with her father, her daughter would be away for several Thursdays and she would be able to attend the group after all.

The following week we were working on painting masks and she immediately turned her mask over and painted the interior first (see Figures 2.5 and 2.6). This meant that, unlike that of her peers, her artwork on her mask was not visible to others as she worked. In fact, as she worked, she held the mask up like a wall between us. Behind this wall, she painted with quiet concentration. When it was complete, she called me over to show me its dark interior and talked about the emotions she struggled with. As she did so, she began to cry, and again left the room immediately. During our group processing, a peer asked her to share about her mask, commenting on her method of pouring the paint on to allow it to create the drip pattern on the exterior. Elle did indeed share her mask with the group, crying as she talked about the emotional weight it depicted and the way in which she struggles with that. She did not leave the room, and she was met with an outpouring of support from members young and old. Her emotional discussion led others to discuss some of their more difficult struggles with re-entering civilian life, coping with injury and more. An older gentleman who had only started attending a few weeks prior stated that he was a Vietnam veteran who finally acknowledged that he needed help with PTSD and related symptoms one year ago. Another shared that he related to her mask and felt as if neither his family nor the VA saw him beneath his mask. In this way, she received support directly, but also witnessed that she was not the only one struggling with her emotional recovery.

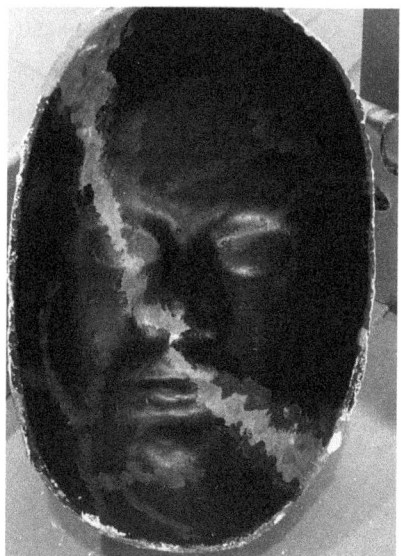

Figure 2.5: Interior of Elle's mask

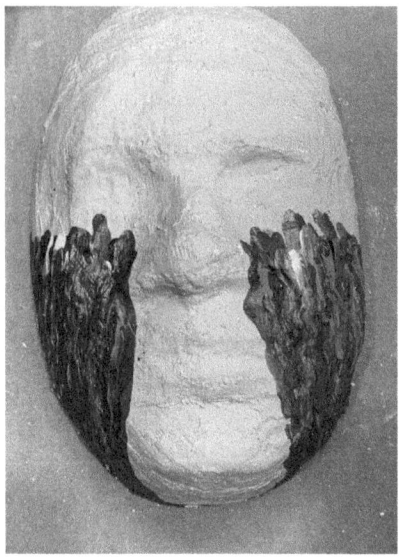

Figure 2.6: Exterior of Elle's mask

The discussion, and some of the comments Elle made, particularly about female veterans, led the group to identify two potential new projects. One of her points during the discussion was how hurtful it feels when she is out with male veterans and they are thanked for their service, but she is overlooked and assumed to be a military spouse rather than a veteran herself. This led the group to discuss how different they all were in appearance, whether in gender, race, or age, and with visible disabilities or not. They began to explore the possibility of placing a large group photo at our next art exhibit and inviting viewers to see if they could "spot the veteran" to drive home the fact that there is no one version of a veteran. In fact, the punchline would be that everyone in the photograph would be a veteran. At the time of this writing, talks are underway to reach out to some veterans' social groups for participation in this photography project.

IMPACT ON ISOLATION VERSUS
SOCIAL CONNECTION

The group makeup morphs and changes as the months go by, but even with these gradual changes in makeup, there has been a consistent trend of increasing cohesion. While not easily quantified, this is observable in comments that indicate that group members are making social connections and contacting each other outside the group sessions, and in comments shared during focus group discussions. This suggests the group is meeting a need for social connection that could be combating the isolation often cited as a concern for veterans who must leave the camaraderie of their military peers in active service and re-enter civilian life. When asked why he chose to start attending, one of the longest-running members of the group, said simply, "I figured, hey, it's a chance to get out of the house one night a week." Another member followed up with a similar comment, stating, "I'm an isolator, so if it wasn't for the class I'd probably be at home also."

I have observed a group member giving a peer (whom she had not known prior to their time in this group together) a ride to the group so she would not miss the session. I have seen bonds that deepen into the type of friendship where group members greet each other with hugs. For a brief period, veterans' families were participating alongside them in the group, including children, and such a rapport was created that one group member arrived one week with a present for the child of another member.

The group itself often becomes a powerful healing force. The connection with others serves to combat isolation as described above and by extension can mitigate the related depression. Meeting with others in a somewhat social setting—which the group has thanks to its snacks, coffee, and occasional trips down to evening receptions in the gallery—can also reintroduce pleasurable experiences and emotions to those who may have forgotten or foregone them. Art making in a group setting doubles up on this by providing socialization and a pleasant activity (Collie *et al.*, 2006).

IMPACT ON COMMUNITY CONNECTION

The museum extends a complimentary museum membership to all veterans, and regular and personalized invitations to Art for Warriors' participants to partake in special events affiliated with the museum. The group meets on Thursday evenings which is also often the evening of artists' receptions for the museum's changing exhibits. Group members regularly join the receptions on the way upstairs to group or on their way out following group. During these events, they can try on yet another role, that of art lover or patron. They mingle with another subset of their larger community and strike another blow against isolation and the avoidance or inability to enjoy pleasurable experiences they may have been struggling with. Their art making is inspired and fed by this process of viewing new artwork, and the entire endeavor of art making is legitimized.

Veterans become comfortable with the museum and are often recognized and warmly welcomed by staff. The institution transforms in their perception from something distant and removed to a place of great familiarity. It becomes a resource for leisure and recreation and is added to their arsenal of coping skills as another viable way to combat limited social outlets. They can not only participate in the group but also take classes with a members' discount. Indeed, periodically we partner with the museum's instructors to bring in more direct instruction and a higher level of technical expertise. This has led to successful forays into the ceramics studio, new skills in landscape painting and unique opportunities to partake in public art projects. At the museum, the veterans take on new roles as artist and patron.

The museum has a close working relationship with the city and therefore community events outside the museum are also highlighted and announced to the veterans. While these are often social and recreational in nature, at times more meaningful opportunities are afforded them. The Power of Art project is one such opportunity. Power of Art is a two-year project bringing a series of five temporary public art projects to the cities of Coral Springs and Parkland to aid in the healing and community rebuilding needed in the aftermath of the school shooting at Marjorie Stoneman Douglas (MSD) High School. The museum is just a few minutes from MSD, and approximately half of MSD students are actually residents of Coral Springs, not neighboring Parkland. As a result, the entire community felt the ripples of that act of violence, including members of our Art for Warriors program. Community involvement is a key component of each of the five public art projects, and due to the museum's direct participation in the creation and planning of the Power of Art projects, the art therapy group members have received wonderful direct access to work alongside the artists. For the first event, artist David Best (of Burning Man) fame came to Coral Springs to construct one of his beautiful temples. Art for Warriors was one of a limited number of community groups invited to design a panel for inclusion in the temple (Figure 2.7). One of the Art for Warriors members gave so much of his time and construction expertise to the artist and his crew that he was invited to join them on future builds in other cities. Overall, experiences like this provide powerful ways for veterans to be recognized and included in their larger communities and can help them reconnect to the places they live. These events and endeavors defy isolation and disinterest because they involve social interaction, collaboration, and pleasurable activities.

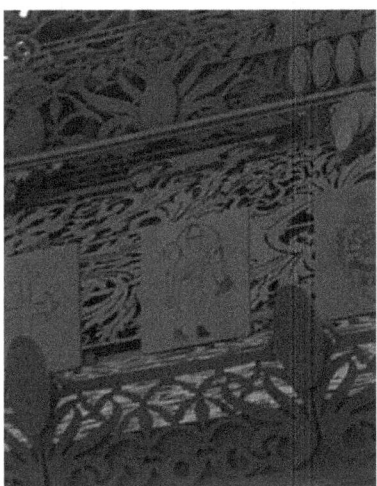

Figure 2.7: Art for Warriors panel designed for the Power of Art Temple

IMPACT ON STRESS, COPING SKILLS, AND LEISURE

Participants in the group receive didactic information on stress management tools such as deep breathing and progressive muscle relaxation, sometimes going so far as written handouts. They also receive a written resource sheet that includes national crisis lines, veteran-specific providers and referral services, and local resources. This information is provided in writing in the form a resource sheet or pamphlet that is displayed each week. Copies are made available each week for participants. In this way, they are guaranteed to at least be aware of and introduced to a variety of stress-management techniques.

The role of art and art making is also discussed often. Participants can reflect on how attending the group and working on their art impacts their mood and energy each week thanks to our check-in and check-out. By rating their overall mood and energy on a general scale from 0 to 10 at the beginning and end of each group they can observe whether, as has proven to be the case, they are leaving with a higher rating than when they came in. Participating in the group also provides them with first-hand experience in the ways social interaction and connections with others can provide them with support and be its own coping skill. In addition, as one of the members recently pointed out during a discussion, not only can it be helpful to receive support from their peers, it can also be equally important to feel they are being "of service to other veterans" by being part of this group.

CONCLUSIONS AND CONSIDERATIONS

Veterans face a myriad of challenges reacclimating to civilian life, and the impact of serving and of leaving military life can be long-lasting and complex. The literature suggests that art therapy is effective at dealing with many of the precise symptoms and challenges faced by returning veterans. A program that finds ways to reduce stigma, remove obstacles such as cost, and make participation and eligibility easy and accessible can be an effective way to reach a wide audience of veterans. Being based within an art museum provides Art for Warriors with unique resources that enrich the art therapy experience for veterans. These include not only material resources such as grant funding to facilitate the program and works of art, but social resources such as community events and artists' receptions.

For those wishing to establish something similar, I offer some points to consider. It is advised that you set specific parameters at the beginning of your group about who will be considered eligible. For example, is the group restricted to veterans only or will it be open to spouses? Art for Warriors has decreasing isolation as one of its goals, and allowing spouses to attend can directly contribute to decreasing isolation that veterans often feel from civilians in their lives. However, if you allow spouses, will you allow children? Of what age? A program for veterans and their children will require different materials and different topics than a group without children, and you will want to set those guidelines early. Consider any restrictions from your funding source, as well as the goals of the program and the needs of your participants when deciding on participant eligibility. For example, will you be required to confirm their veteran status and, if so, how? In the case of our program, we do this with a simple questionnaire that asks people to identify their branch and years of service, but some programs may require more official documentation or even screen for specific presenting problems or diagnoses.

In terms of determining who will be eligible to participate, I offer the following anecdote for your consideration. One evening, as it so happened, no spouses or adult children of veterans showed up for group. We had, instead, a small group of older males. During their greetings and introductions, a couple of them realized they had served in the same conflict. As they compared notes with each other, the conversation turned to their experiences on their return. A quarter of the group time passed in this way, with the men connecting with each other, even with those from different conflicts, about these difficult experiences. Feeling pressure to get the group on to an art therapy directive, I attempted to segue the discussion into an art project. They paused their conversation and listened politely as I attempted to find a foothold in the conversation that would allow us to transition to art making, and as soon as I was done describing the art making directive, they promptly resumed their conversation. We passed almost the entire two hours of group time in this way. One member in particular talked more and shared in greater detail about personally difficult aspects of his return from combat than he ever had before, despite months of attendance. It remains to this day one of the most impactful and revelatory discussions of a difficult topic the group has ever had. Though one can never know for certain what prompts such an experience, and I suspect it is a combination of ingredients that spark the magic of those times when a group just really seems to click, I wonder if it was related to the homogeneity of the group's attendees that night and the permission to speak without their spouses or family members hearing what they had to say.

Consider also what the mechanism will be for publicizing the group. We have found that it is necessary to do this on an ongoing basis, and despite being in existence for three years, we still have new attendees who say, "I never knew this was here!" You cannot help veterans in your community if they do not know you are there, so this is key to your mission. Try contacting area VA hospitals and facilities, veterans' coalitions, student veteran organizations, non-profits that provide support services to veterans, and be sure reach out to your community's first responders as many of them are often veterans.

It is also important to consider funding and how you plan to measure the impact of your program. These two factors go hand in hand. Funders will want to know what your goals are as well as how you plan to measure whether they have been achieved. Clearly delineate the scope of responsibilities for the art therapist, as well as for the partnering agency. Program evaluation for funding purposes can be different from the standards art therapists may be accustomed to for research purposes and it is important to know the difference.

The art therapy and art museum partnership can help the museum with the audience outreach and service to community members that are its goals. The art therapist can benefit from access to the museum's objects, expertise, aesthetic, and physical space. Participants benefit when they have a less stigmatizing place where they can receive support and form connections. In these ways, I see art therapists' goals, art museums' missions, and community members' needs naturally intersecting and dovetailing. Despite the potential benefits to all involved, these types of alliances remain an uncommon approach to art therapy programming for veterans, but it is my hope that this chapter will help to change that.

Chapter 3

Hand-Papermaking with Student Veterans

— MEREDITH MCMACKIN —

INTRODUCTION

In this chapter I share my personal journey that led me to work with
veterans and become an art therapist. I describe how I learned about
the therapeutic process of hand-papermaking with student veterans and
share my initial hands-on experiences of making paper from military
uniforms. Witnessing this transformative process led to the decision to
focus my research on papermaking with student veterans. The following
is a summary of my dissertation: *Assessing the Value of Creative Arts
Workshops and Hand Papermaking for Student Veterans in Transition*
(McMackin, 2016).

This journey began with the death of my older son, who was killed
in combat while on his second deployment in Iraq. Following his death,
I kept looking for something meaningful I could do with my life in
response to this loss. As an artist, I used art making as an outlet and a
way to express the grief that was hard to put into words. But I wanted
to do more. I kept thinking that I wanted to do something to help bring
more peace to our planet, but I didn't know what that might be.

Working as an academic advisor at a large university in the south-
eastern United States, I was offered the opportunity to advise the student
veteran organization on campus. I felt a deep satisfaction with this work

and a real connection to these students, many of whom were combat veterans. Because of hearing stories of my son's military experiences, I could relate to their stories and I had some idea of their difficulties. I hoped that by supporting warriors in their healing process, perhaps I could help bring more peace to this planet. This work is my way to honor my son's life and service and to support his fellow service members who have given so much.

UNDERSTANDING STUDENT VETERAN ISSUES AND PREVIOUS RESEARCH

The Iraq and Afghanistan-era war veterans make up the largest population of combat veterans since the Vietnam War (Vespa, 2020). With increased benefits for education included in the post 9/11 GI Bill (Molina, 2014; Vespa, 2020), a growing number of recently discharged veterans are choosing to attend college. Recognizing the challenges facing this transition, colleges and universities have made efforts to increase programs and services to support veterans through multiple adjustments (DiRamio & Jarvis, 2011). Additionally, this population includes a significant percentage of student veterans dealing with disabilities, both seen and unseen (Thomas *et al.*, 2010). Recent studies related to military and veteran cultures include issues such as, but not limited to, post-traumatic stress disorder (PTSD) and traumatic brain injury (TBI), often referred to as the "signature injuries" (Hoge, 2010, p.2) of the wars in Iraq and Afghanistan.

My own experience has taught me that student veterans have many differences from average college students. They are an older population with life experiences that students who came straight from high school cannot even imagine. There can be a social disconnect with younger, non-veteran students who, in turn, may have difficulty relating to a veteran's military experiences. Veterans may also be supporting families and have additional responsibilities demanding their time outside school. Student veterans must also learn to manage multiple bureaucracies for school funding and healthcare.

Multiple studies have shown art therapy to be successful in providing support to veterans in both individual and group settings, enabling veterans to process and externalize traumatic memories (Canto *et al.*, 2015; Collie *et al.*, 2006; Kopytin & Lebedev, 2013; Lobban, 2014; Mims, 2015). Visual journaling with student veterans showed an increased expression of self-knowledge and more self-confidence in their ability to express themselves through art making (Mims, 2015). Canto *et al.'s* 2015 study with student veterans found that arts workshops provided an opportunity to externalize difficult memories and allow participants to share their stories with each other and the university community.

INTRODUCTION TO THE THERAPEUTIC USE OF HAND-PAPERMAKING

In 2012 I attended a large event in the greater Washington DC area called "The Arts, Military, and Healing Initiative" and I participated in a workshop facilitated by the Peace Paper Project. I had heard of Combat Paper and the Peace Paper Project and was thrilled to have an opportunity to experience the process. This was my first experience of making paper with student veterans and I witnessed the transformative process of using their uniforms and personal images in creating handmade paper works of art.

As I observed veterans and military family members making paper from discarded uniforms, I used left-over sections of a Marine uniform and thought about my son. I cut the uniform into small pieces, in preparation for adding it to the Hollander Beater. Learning to use the traditional papermaking hand tools of the mould and deckle, I felt the excitement and fascination of transforming the uniform into a unique, new piece of paper art.

As I had shared my experience with the veterans center director of the university I was attending, the Peace Paper Project was invited to provide a workshop at our student veterans center. Over the next several years, the center sponsored the Peace Paper Project annually, eventually leading to the center purchasing its own equipment and supplies for a mobile papermaking studio. I witnessed veteran after veteran experience the meaningful and literal transformation of remnants of their military memories into expressive art, and I saw both the fun and excitement along with quiet times of reflection.

FORMULATING MY DOCTORAL RESEARCH

My own experience participating in several papermaking workshops with student veterans led me to realize that I had never experienced such a meaningful therapeutic art process and powerful group experience. Because of the impact from my own experience and observing the participants' responses, I chose this subject for my doctoral research. The research design and findings will be detailed later in this chapter.

After the previous papermaking workshops at the university, there had been very little follow-up or organized gathering of response data from the participants. I wanted to learn more about their individual experiences of meaning-making and how it might have facilitated the participants' transition to college, and to understand the impact of the human connections and friendships that were formed through the shared experience. I also hoped to validate the importance and need for special programs for veterans in higher education.

STUDIES USING ART THERAPY
WITH COMBAT VETERANS

After reviewing multiple studies by art therapists working with combat veterans suffering from PTSD, Collie *et al.* (2006) found that the best results in group art therapy were where veterans had established trust and empathy for one another. Art became symbolic objects that provided emotional distance and helped the participants externalize memories. The authors also noted that the visual arts gave veterans the ability to create non-verbal, visual narratives of traumatic experiences, reconsolidate memories, and place troubling memories in the past. Their participants reported that the process of art making was relaxing and enjoyable, which encouraged positive emotions, and gave the veterans a sense of self-efficacy.

In Lobban's studies of the functioning of the brain (2014), she found that the areas of the brain that control language are affected by trauma, indicating that the effects of PTSD can cause suppression of verbal language. At the same time, she found evidence of increased activity in the right hemisphere, an area associated with visual imagery and emotions. Through her experiences using art therapy in a center for veterans with PTSD, Lobban shared how art making gave veterans an opportunity to communicate non-verbally and to visually express suppressed and unconscious thoughts, feelings, and memories. To avoid trauma-affected veterans isolating themselves, Lobban stressed the importance of group work to develop trusting relationships and a sense of community. Having a sense of safety among other veterans made it easier to process traumatic memories that emerged through their art.

PHILOSOPHICAL AND THEORETICAL APPROACH TO RESEARCH

Using qualitative methods, I chose phenomenology as my philosophical stance in my dissertation research because of my interest in individual perception and how we give meaning to the phenomenon we experience (Husserl, 1952; Merleau-Ponty, 2012). My dissertation examined how the papermaking workshop facilitated the transition for student veterans and how they interpreted their life experiences through the creative arts. Mala Betensky (2001) wrote about her phenomenological approach to meaning-making through art. She believed that art is self-expression from the core of one's being, and that through conscious looking and reflection clients would begin to discover meaningful insights.

Symbolic interactionism, a social science theory (Becker & McCall, 1990; Blumer, 1969), was used as a conceptual framework in assessing how the group interactions affected the individual experiences of the papermaking workshop participants. This research also provided further insight into the individual challenges of student veterans in their transition from the military into college. Additionally, I also considered theories related to adult transitions (Schlossberg, 2011), human agency and self-efficacy (Benight & Bandura, 2004), self-authorship in education (Baxter-Magolda, 2007), and meaning-making (Frankel, 1959).

My research gave me an opportunity to observe, interview, and document individual experiences and the impact the workshop had on student veterans' transition and adjustment into the university after leaving the military. Based on past experience, I believed that being a part of the group would provide greater access to the participants and foster the development of relationships through shared experiences. As facilitator, I assisted as needed in the studio, demonstrated art-making processes, and sometimes created artwork along with the participants. Being actively involved helped me get acquainted with the workshop attendees, and it was also a way of gaining trust and developing a sense of comfort and ease in their interactions. This allowed me to refrain from creating distance between researcher and the participants by unobtrusively observing participant interactions.

THE PARTICIPANT SAMPLE

The participants were recruited through the student veterans center at the university. In addition to speaking to groups about the workshop, I had the support from the director and staff of the veterans center as well as student veterans who had participated in previous workshops at the university. Although more had signed up, a total of six veterans participated in the workshop; this included four male and two female student veterans. One was a Marine, four were Army veterans, and one had served in the Navy. Two were graduate students. All but one had deployed overseas, and four had direct combat experience. Three were married and three had children. For three, it was their first year at the university.

PARTICIPANTS' PRE-WORKSHOP PREPARATIONS

The process of reflecting on their military service began a few weeks before the workshop, when they were asked to consider if they wanted to use one of their own uniforms. They were also asked to choose an image they would print on their paper that related somehow to their experiences. The participants (whose names were changed to maintain confidentiality) all chose to use their own uniforms except for Bart, who used his deceased friend's uniform. They reflected on where they wore their uniforms, which brought back memories of military experience. Each person had different levels of attachment and chose the uniform to cut up and pulp for a variety of reasons. Bryan, a student who participated in part of the workshop the year before, said, "It was actually kinda interesting to pick which one." He said he had "a ton of them" (McMackin, 2016, p.87) but it took a while to choose one he could cut up. Mark said he had worn his uniform in both of his deployments to Afghanistan in 2010 and 2011.

The images the participants chose were made into a silkscreen stencil to print onto their handmade paper before the workshop began. A graphic designer on campus used an illustrator program to transform the images into black and white shapes. Altered images were sent to each of the participants for their approval before exposing the images on the screens. The final simplified stencil-like image was then burned into the light-sensitive emulsion coating on individual pieces of silkscreen fabric.

Reviewing images and reflecting on their military experience was another process that, for some, uncovered memories that elicited strong emotions. Participants had to choose an image they felt was especially significant to print on the paper made from their own uniform, or in Bart's case, his deceased best friend's. Bryan explained that he chose an image related to a friend who was killed during their first deployment in 2008. The photograph was taken recently when he and his family attended a memorial for his friend and others. In his final interview, he shared the significance of the image, stating:

> It was a few months ago, there was a reunion for my old unit that I
> deployed to Iraq with, and so we went up there and I took the entire

family, and the picture is of my son pointing at the name of the guy who his middle name is for, on the memorial wall that is actually getting torn down. There's an initiative to save it but, it's not going too well…but yeah, that was really cool, I pointed to it first and said you know that's the name of the guy you were named after and right after I pointed at it, he pointed at it too. (McMackin, 2016, pp.90–91)

THE PAPERMAKING WORKSHOP

The workshop took place in the art department's sculpture lab at the university. We were fortunate to have the space to ourselves most of the weekend. We used the large table in the main open lab area for the initial introductions and as a uniform cutting table; this also became the social gathering area and where we ate lunch. We set out cutting mats, scissors, and rolling blade cutters around the table, with stools for students to sit on. The table was high enough to work on while standing up as well.

Background and introductions

I began the workshop by introducing myself and my journey to becoming an art therapist, working with student veterans, and being inspired by my son's service and giving his life in Iraq. I shared my personal information because I wanted them to understand my connection to the military. I described the format of the workshop as using "art as therapy" rather than "art therapy," explaining that I would be emphasizing the therapeutic benefits inherent in the creative act of making art itself without requiring verbal processing and analysis with a therapist.

A history of veteran papermaking workshops at the university was explained, including the process of making paper from uniforms, which was originally introduced to student veterans by the Peace Paper Project. Lastly, I gave a brief introduction of the history of hand-papermaking, beginning in China in 105AD (Hunter, 1978) and traveling through the Middle East, specifically Bagdad, and then spreading through the Muslim world to reach Europe and the Western world. I thought that making the historical connection of papermaking to Iraq and the Muslim world might be meaningful to the veterans who had served there.

I then asked each of the participants to share a little about themselves. They were asked to talk about their background in the military, where they served, their experience of separating from the military, and what brought them to this university. I also asked them to share what sparked their interest in participating in the workshop.

Bryan was in the Army from 2000–2010. He said he wasn't really interested in academia in high school and that was one of the reasons he joined the Army. However, he shared that after leaving the military he became inspired to try to make it to university after seeing the university student veteran group marching in the Veterans Day parade. Also, his father was an alumni, he grew up in the town, and was a big a fan of the school and the football team. He shared a story about one of his best friends who was killed by a roadside bomb in Iraq in 2008. He said:

> He was just kind of a memory that lived with me…so I decided that for one, I was going to make the paper for myself out of my own uniform, cuz it's cool to do a physical transition of something that was with me all the time, on my body all the time and then turn it into something I can display on my wall at home. So I thought that was really neat and then I realized, hey, I could send a really cool image on this paper to his family as a way of saying, hey I've been thinking about him since 2008 and you know, he won't be forgotten. (McMackin, 2016, p.101)

The workshop gave him the opportunity to externalize the memory of his friend and create a symbolic object to honor his friend and to share with others.

Learning to make paper

After the introductions, I led the group through to the sculpture lab to show them the space and demonstrate the process of papermaking. We walked to the covered outside area and I introduced the participants to the Hollander Beater, the machine that breaks down the cloth to fiber (see Figure 3.1). Bryan was the first to pulp his uniform and he added the pieces a little at a time, pushing them down so they were immersed in the water and would circulate through the blades. The steel blades attach to a heavy steel cylinder. When the machine is switched on, the cylinder begins to turn, which makes the water in the trough circulate. As you stand and watch, the small scraps of cloth circle through the beater blades, you see the fibers loosen and after a while (30 minutes to an hour generally), it turns to pulp, unrecognizable anymore as a uniform.

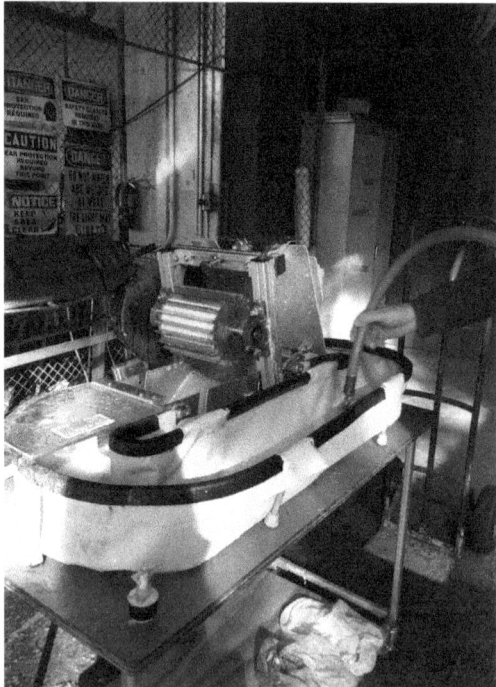

Figure 3.1: The Hollander Beater that is used to turn cloth into fiber for hand-papermaking

Next, the participants were led into an adjacent enclosed room, which also connected to the large lab area where we began the group. This smaller room had four tables with two large plastic trays on each table and a plywood board beside each tray (see Figure 3.2). It was explained that this was the "sheet formation" area and a demonstration was given showing how a sheet of paper is formed out of the pulp. An immediate process of transferring an image onto the freshly pressed paper (known as "pulp printing") was then demonstrated.

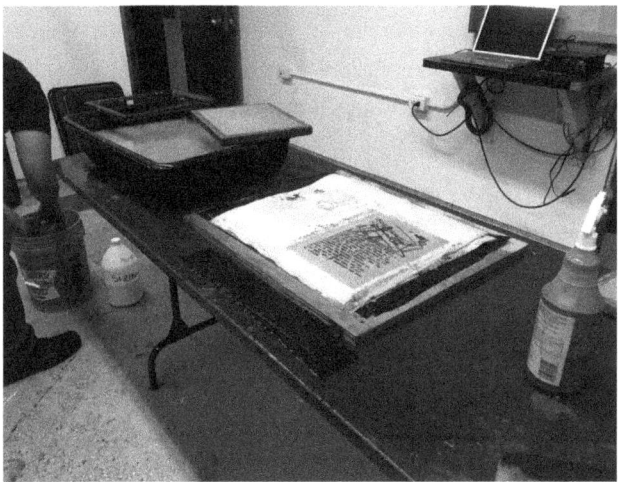

Figure 3.2: Table setup for hand-papermaking

Once all of the stages of the process had been demonstrated, the participants were told that they could start cutting their uniform and I and the volunteers would be around to help if they needed anything. They were instructed to cut the fabric into little squares, approximately the size of a postage stamp. This can be an emotional process, with participants reflecting on memories associated with the uniform. I referred to this as the deconstruction phase of the process.

I was pleasantly surprised when Kenneth, a student veteran and papermaking veteran, arrived. He had gone through training to assist with papermaking workshops the year before. Kenneth had a warm smile and greeted those he knew in the room, and was introduced to the new students. He visited with the others most of the time but later helped students individually if they needed assistance in the sheet formation process. Everyone seemed very relaxed and appeared to be enjoying themselves. I was pleased as I had hoped to provide the atmosphere and looseness of former workshops, which I felt would help relieve any anxiety or stress about the process.

At this point, students were working at their own pace, and the conversations began to flow. Bryan, who was waiting for his pulp to finish, sat and joined in with the conversations. There was plenty of laughter and joking around. Then something would come up about their military experiences and they shared more stories. There was a kind of balance between small talk and memories that related to their experiences in the military and in war, which kept the atmosphere in the room from feeling too emotionally heavy. Mark, Bart, and Kenneth were talking about different areas they were stationed in during their deployments to Iraq and Afghanistan. Mark made a comment about someone he knew who had over 100 kills in combat. Having not been in combat, hearing them talk about "kills" in such a seemingly nonchalant manner was disconcerting to me, but I kept my feelings to myself (McMackin, 2016, p.107).

Making social connections was crucial to the success and meaning-making that participants took from the workshop. In the written reflections they wrote at the end of the second day, four out of the five who completed the reflection form mentioned getting to know each other and hearing each other's stories as a meaningful part of the experience. George wrote: "I enjoyed the company of my fellow vets. It was nice to just be in a low stress environment with very cool people" (McMackin, 2016, p.108).

Reflecting on the many comments by the participants on the value of the social aspect of the workshop, I was reminded that military training and culture promotes and instills a sense of community and interdependence within the troops. They leave that sense of family when they leave the military and re-enter civilian culture, which can lead to feelings of isolation. Because most Americans have not served in the military, veterans find themselves part of a minority. Participating in the papermaking workshop gave veterans time to relax in a supportive environment, to connect with fellow veterans and re-establish a kind of community.

During the workshop, while participants were in different phases of the process, the large table in the main room became a social gathering location, the central location for developing "communitas," a term used by Michael Schwalbe (1996) to define the connections fostered through the sense of shared group experience. Bryan recalled a time when the participants were gathered around the table, and the conversation turned to their military past and they spontaneously began to share stories of their experiences. He said: "We hardly knew each other, but we all just kinda opened up and started telling war stories...so it was really cool cuz how we all kinda clicked. Just cuz of a shared experience" (McMackin, 2016, p.109). In the presence of other combat veterans, he knew they could relate.

Deconstruction

For some, the most challenging part of the process was seemingly destroying something that symbolized a hugely significant part of their past. For Bryan, it was the hardest thing to do, but he described it as the most "therapeutic" part of the papermaking process. At first he was skeptical about cutting his uniform, thinking, "I can't believe I'm cutting up a piece of my history," and he re-emphasized that, "like I said, I was really attached to all of those pieces." But as he was cutting his uniform, he was convincing himself it would be okay, and he told himself, "This is going to be something that I can hold onto and it will be even more meaningful" (McMackin, 2016, p.111). He realized that it was also a kind of release, a letting go of the past and said, "I'm shredding up a piece of something that I've been holding on to" (p.111). Listening to him took me back to my own experience with papermaking, having pulped the dress I bought to wear to my son's memorial service. I had felt a mixture of feelings, but knowing I didn't want to wear the dress again made it easier. When I began cutting my dress, images and memories flooded my mind. Figure 3.3 shows how small a piece of fabric must be cut in order to use it for papermaking.

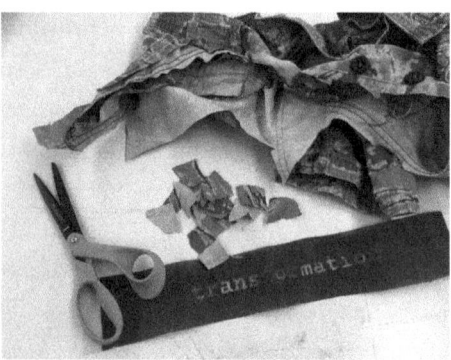

Figure 3.3: A military uniform being cut up for hand-papermaking

Mark, who got a later start than the others, was sometimes working alone at the table while others were in different areas involved in various stages of the making process. He said he remembered all of the things that happened to him when he was wearing that uniform while in Afghanistan. He was trying to let go of some of those memories, the "hard, fearful feelings and scary feelings and feeling of disappointment" (McMackin, 2016, p.111), and put them in the past. He said he told himself, "It's done and it's over with and nothing can change from the past" (p.111). In his individual interview several weeks later, he said, "It was a way for me to let go of my memories that I had of what I had gone through and what I had done while I was deployed and to let it go was like a weight being lifted off my chest" (p.111).

George said he had been drawn to the idea of using the uniforms. He used the terms "recycling" and "repurposing" (McMackin, 2016, p.112) and saw it as symbolic of the process of reinventing oneself after leaving the military. He connected the transformation of the uniform to the life changes veterans go through. The physical process made an impact on him, as he explained:

> Seeing something that had a very specific purpose and then rebuilding it into something that has a different purpose, it's kind of what a lot of us are doing as we transition out of the military. It's kind of repurposing our lives because our lives have been built around doing one particular

thing whatever that thing happens to be, because being in the military is not really a job so much as it's an entire way of life. So now I'm doing something else, it's kind of like you're remaking yourself, you're recycling your whole mindset I guess. (McMackin, 2016, p.112)

Reconstruction

Sheet formation involves whole body movement, with repetitive motion that is slow and smooth. Although they had seen the demonstration and watched others making paper, it took a few attempts for the students to get comfortable with the process. However, it is easy to start over, as the pulp can always be returned back into the tub of water, and then you can try it again (see Figure 3.4). Once the paper was pressed, the participants had the option of printing their own or other images onto the wet surface of the paper, or to leave some sheets without images. The amount of paper each participant made varied from 12 to 35 sheets.

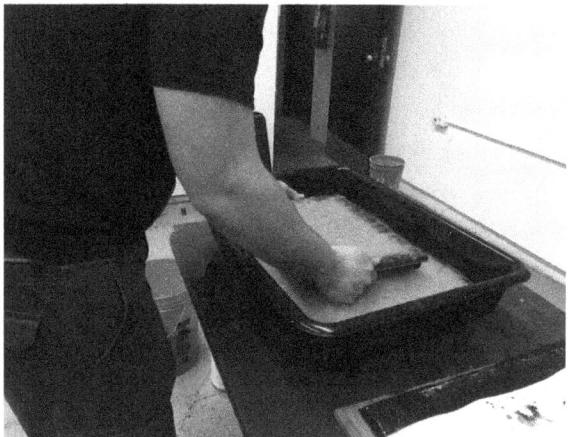

Figure 3.4: A workshop participant makes sheets of paper

During the process of pulp printing, there were moments of uncertainty, not knowing what the image would look like until the stencil was removed. Some were clean and well defined, and at other times, the image was blurred and smudged. The excitement was contagious, watching the participants delight in how the image looked on the paper.

There was a learning curve, and at times it could be frustrating. Bart expressed the frustration he felt in the beginning and the pressure because, as he stated, "it was for me but it was also for, you know, my friend's family" (McMackin, 2016, p.115). He said that it was something that takes practice. The more paper he made and printing he did, the more he began to relax into the process. He said he wasn't an "artist person" so at first the imperfections made him nervous but then he realized "it kind of creates character I guess in the piece" (p.115). By the end of the workshop, each participant was able to experience success and had created multiple sheets with prints as well as blank sheets.

At the end of each day we sandwiched each participant's stack of paper on pellon sheets (also known as interfacing) between thick plywood boards and gathered together to create what is affectionately known as a "people press," to press out as much water as possible before hanging up the pellon sheets to dry (see Figure 3.5). Someone found a large, heavy medal grate in the area so that even more people could stand on the boards at once. About five to six people stepped up onto the grate and everyone held onto each other for balance. There was a lot of laughter and people taking photos with their phones. Once the water had been squeezed out of the paper stacks, everyone helped hang the pellon sheets with the attached wet paper to clothes lines that had been strung across the sheet formation room.

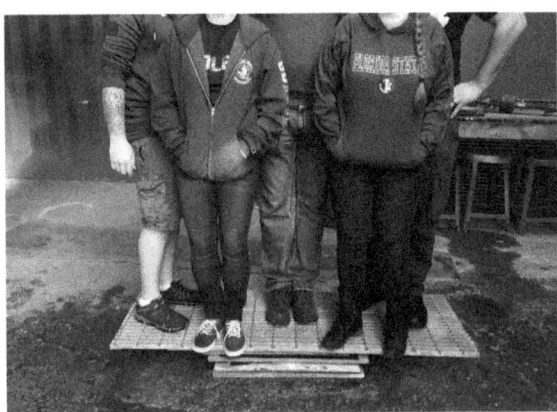

Figure 3.5: Workshop participants using a people press to help dry pellon sheets

Follow up and exhibit

A week or so later, I met with the participants at a social gathering in the veterans center and gave them their paper after it was dried and pressed smooth and flat using a paper press. They were asked to pick out one piece that they would like to have framed for an exhibit of their work to be displayed in the main school library. Each veteran wrote a statement which was to be displayed on the wall next to their framed artwork. They were also asked if they would like to donate one piece for the new veteran handmade paper archive that was started by the special collections department of the university library. Some, but not all, gave one piece they wanted to contribute and wrote a short statement about the paper and the image.

The final event was several weeks after the workshop. The time lapse was intended to give participants time to reflect on the experience as well as time to frame, organize, and hang the exhibit. Seeing their work framed and hung in the university library after a period of time gave them a fresh look at their work, allowing them to view it as a work of art and worthy of a public exhibition.

After having one piece for each participant professionally framed, we had an opening reception which was advertised around campus. There was a short opening talk and several people spoke, including me, one of the workshop participants, and the director of the veterans center. The message was one of celebrating the work and the value of sharing their personal stories with the university community. It was a message of inclusion, again strengthening the sense of family and communitas.

Invoking pride, inclusion, and connection

All of the student veterans expressed the pride they felt in having their work hanging in the library. The main university library was a kind of central hub for students at the university, many of whom pass through on a daily basis. The work was hung in the main entrance and in front of the check-out counter. In the interview following the opening, Bart expressed his pride when he talked about how much it meant to him to be a student at the university. He said, "I'm very proud to have it hanging up in Strozier. I'm very proud to be here to begin with, so like being a (university) student, like it means as much to me as being a Marine" (McMackin, 2016, p.121). He also said, "I'm very proud you know, to represent my friend and his life and being a Marine, somewhere where people will appreciate it" (p.121).

The opening exhibit was emotional for Bryan. He brought his oldest son with him and when his son saw the image and read what his dad had written about his friend's death, the seven-year-old's eyes filled with tears. As Bryan was telling me about his son's reaction in the individual interview a few days later, his emotions spilled over. The impact on Bryan was intensified because his older son was so affected by the death of his dad's friend and seemed to comprehend the connection with his little brother, who had been named after the friend. The piece Bryan selected for the exhibit can be seen in Figure 3.6.

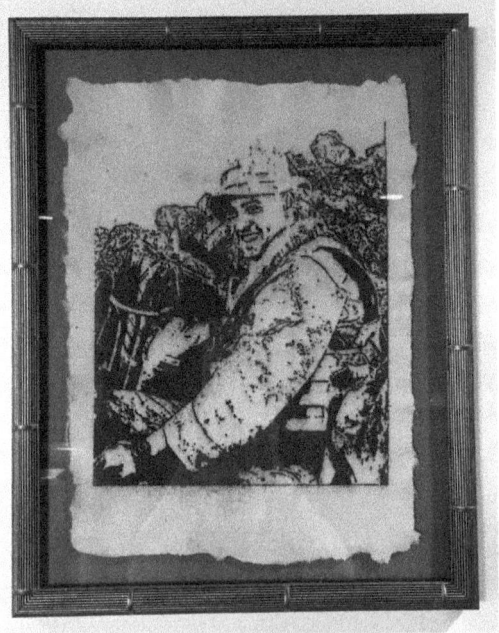

Figure 3.6: Bryan's art depicting his fallen comrade

Having the exhibit in the university library not only filled the participants with pride, it connected them with the university in a powerful way. They shared the stories from their military experience with the students and staff of the school, who responded enthusiastically. The exhibition organizer wrote several weeks later, saying, "Many guests commented on the individual pieces and shared their personal stories of their military experiences or those of their family members" (McMackin, 2016, p.124). Bart said, "Being able to share stories with everyone was pretty key in my opinion. Like that was really neat" (p.124).

Having their art as a reminder

Long after the workshop and the exhibit ended, the participants still have the art as a reminder of the experience. Most have kept their work. Some perhaps hung the framed print in their house. Others gave their work as a gift to family members or close friends. The art is a tangible reminder of the creative experience as well as their military service. A few months after the workshop, Amanda's grandfather, whose image she had printed on her paper, passed away. She contacted me to say that her grandmother placed the framed handmade paper image next to her grandfather's casket at his memorial service and her mother mentioned her piece during the service. Amanda was touched to hear about the impact of her work and the ripple effect it had on her family.

Process of analysis and emergent themes

In my analysis of my data collected through observation, written statements, and recorded interviews, I noted key words and statements participants made in relation to their experiences, past and present. I began to see common themes between multiple sources that emerged from the data. Prominent themes included: redefining the self; the significance of sharing stories and connecting with others; developing mutual support and communitas; balancing emotions with activities and social engagement; meaning-making; self-reflection and emotional processing from past experiences; and invoking institutional pride.

Several participants talked about the workshop helping them let go of some of the negative feelings and painful memories. The deconstruction and transformative processes of making paper from their uniforms created a new way of looking at the experience. Barbara said that the process reminded her of some of the positive memories she had, despite all of the painful ones that often overshadowed the others. She said, "Sometimes even the bad stuff has its own beauty to it. I learned to try to think of the positives" (McMackin, 2016, p.123).

Mark said art was "definitely a way to let off steam" (McMackin, 2016, p.124). He said it had given him time to reflect on what he had done with his life and he was able to open up to other student veterans in the workshop. He said being able to "swap stories" with others "helps relieve stress and it helps relieve some depression and anxiety" (p.124).

Bryan talked about making the print of his friend and how it gave him "some closure" because he was able to create his own memorial; and he said, "There's satisfaction in that I was able to give something for him" (McMackin, 2016, p.124). Besides that, he said he was friends with a couple of other participants before the workshop, but this gave him a chance to get to know them better. It reminded him that he isn't the only one that has experienced war and said it was reassuring to be "with a bunch of people that have been through something pretty similar and you're not the only one" (p.124).

All of the participants learned something new. Several expressed not knowing what to expect, but they all seemed to find lessons they could apply to their lives. Learning to be more patient with themselves, remembering how calming art making could be to them, and realizing that they were creative and capable of making beautiful art were all validating experiences. They gained a greater sense of self-efficacy through their accomplishments and were proud of their work.

CONCLUSION

This chapter describes my journey in sharing the therapeutic use of hand-papermaking with veterans, focusing on my research with student veterans. Through in-depth investigation into the experience of each participant and their interactions, my study found common themes that made the process meaningful and helpful. The participants acknowledged that the papermaking process involving deconstructing military uniforms and repurposing the fibers into handmade paper art was symbolic of their experience of transitioning out of the military and finding a new sense of purpose and identity. They also affirmed that the art they created helped to communicate the meaning of their military service. Finally, connecting with others on campus and having their work recognized by non-veteran students increased their sense of inclusion and support on campus as well as their sense of self-efficacy through learning a new skill and having their work appreciated as an art form. I believe the findings gave validation to the role of the arts as a tool to help veterans transitioning from the military into college. The study also showed how the creative arts can provide veterans with a powerful means to share their stories and increase understanding and communication across campus.

Chapter 4

Building Hope, Resilience, and Freedom in an Open Studio Group

JASHLEY BOATWRIGHT

When veterans feel disenfranchised, isolated, and secluded, art therapy can provide a safe refuge of hope and increase resilience through an open studio art therapy support group. Cathartic breakthroughs eventuate when veterans open themselves up to the art therapy process and begin to heal through trust, vulnerability, feeling safe, and connecting to other veterans. This chapter will explore how veteran art therapy groups can provide a safe container for expression and supportive connection when explosive outbursts and triggers occur.

Research on art therapy with veterans continues to evolve and expand as more and more veterans come back from combat and out of service with symptoms of post-traumatic stress disorder (PTSD). Awareness of PTSD symptoms has increased substantially over the past ten years, which has shown a greater need for trauma work with veterans. Research has shown that art therapy provides a safe place for war-zone content and triggering images to be created and tolerated without complete regression (Johnson, Rosenheck & Fontana, 1997). Art therapy has been shown to be effective in helping veterans transform negative emotions and disturbing images into creative expression

(Jones *et al.*, 2018). Veterans with PTSD who do art therapy have also demonstrated an increase in self-esteem, reconsolidation of memories, improvements in emotional efficacy, and a decline of arousal symptoms (Collie *et al.*, 2006).

The open studio approach to art therapy has long been used across the art therapy field (Allen, 1995, 2005; Moon, 2002). I first learned about this art therapy model when observing groups during my practicum semester for graduate school. Rachel Nash, an Art Institute of Chicago art therapy graduate, was leading these groups. I later had the privilege of co-leading an open studio group for adults experiencing epilepsy with Rachel at her gallery in Dallas, Texas. I fell in love with the intentionality and the creative freedom of the open studio approach, noticing how connection was fostered and expanded as group members increased their confidence in sharing and owning their stories. In an open studio model, the client has ownership and authority over the materials and direction of the artwork.

During this internship, I was placed in the open studio veterans' support group that I now lead. In this group, I was given the honor to learn under Jane Avila, the founder of a non-profit called The Art Station and a pioneer in the art therapy world of north Texas. She had a different perspective of the open studio approach that allowed extensive freedom and choice. She emphasized that the order of introducing art materials was an important progression to familiarity and confidence within the art process. She utilized a Likert scale at the beginning and end of the group for the participants. She also taught me about the importance of meeting the veterans where they were and providing adaptations or extensions to each material if needed. In the first two weeks with new group members, she introduced collage. The following two weeks, veterans got to explore different drawing mediums such as colored pencils, charcoal, oil pastels, drawing pencils, and chalk pastels. Weeks five and six were focused on painting, which often included watercolors and painting with acrylic. Jane reflected on how the military often provides minimal choice and options and instead delivers orders; because of this, she emphasized the importance of choice as a way of empowering the veterans to have the freedom to make their own choices. For the last two weeks, sculpture and clay were introduced, offering considerable opportunities for problem solving. Once veterans completed the progression of art material exposure, they were allowed to create and choose whatever medium they desired.

On my first day as an intern in the veterans' group, I helped a veteran score and hold branches of his clay tree in place as he navigated counterbalancing the weight and depth of his branches. As an intern, I noticed that there were many aspects of the art process that could be triggering for the veterans in the group, such as specific topics centered around politics and the military, and low frustration tolerance with new art mediums. I remember one incident where a veteran who had been a part of the group for two months stormed out of the group and peeled out of the parking lot in his car when he became frustrated with how his art was turning out. Sadly, he never returned to our group. In another situation, the lead therapist appropriately confronted a group member about familial boundaries, which resulted in this veteran never coming back to the group.

After graduation, I was honored to be hired by The Art Station. After a year away from the veterans' group due to other work commitments, I was asked to step into fully leading the group because Jane chose to retire from clinical work. Many of the group members I worked with for a year as an intern were still in the support group. As one can imagine, it was a pivotal and challenging transition from intern to lead therapist. There were many jokes at first within the group reflecting on that transition, but once the dust settled, the veterans in the group were able to acknowledge and accept my new role. I have now had the honor of working with this group for four and a half years.

THE SPACE

Moon (2002) stated that effective art therapy does not have to take place in an idyllic space. The Art Station was previously a fire station and has been re-imagined into an art therapy space with two large rooms and four individual therapy rooms. The open studio space is in a large, rectangular room that once held a fire truck engine. There are two different doors: one that opens to the back hallway and one that opens to the waiting room. The walls are painted a soft, warm yellow and the cabinets are purple and blue. There is natural light shining through seven different windows. The windows are covered on the bottom with a transparent film that allows for privacy while still letting the light in. There is a gallery wall where clients of all ages choose to display their artwork. The studio is full of copious amounts of different art materials, some purchased and some donated. On any given day, one might find anything from wine bottle corks to frames to seashells to glass shards to dolls' hair to donated unused cards to a plethora of fabric. Traditional art therapy materials such as paint (tempera and acrylic), drawing materials (colored pencils, charcoal, pencils, chalk pastels, oil pastels), clay and clay tools, and magazines are also available. Many of the veterans I have worked with compare the space to a "house," describing it "like coming to a home," where they feel safe and invited in. Although the studio room can often get cluttered with donations and overflow with supplies, it is a warm and inviting place full of energy, creativity, and vibrancy.

THE GROUP

The Art Station has led art therapy support groups at the Fort Worth Veterans Affairs (VA) Outpatient Clinic and the University of Arlington. Through a grant with United Way, the group continued at The Art Station, where it has now been meeting for seven years. The grant's lifecycle was completed years ago, but because of Jane's heart and vision for veterans and the great need seen for the program, it has continued to be offered free to veterans even after the grant finished. The Art Station offers two different veteran support groups on different days at different times in the hope of accommodating a variety of schedules; one group meets in the morning and the other in the evening. The groups were originally set as co-ed groups but have naturally evolved into two women's groups. Some of the veterans served in these groups struggle with PTSD, military sexual trauma (MST), traumatic brain injury (TBI), anxiety, depression, and a host of adjustment disorders. PTSD is often comorbid with substance abuse, depression, and anxiety disorders (National Institute of Mental Health, n.d.). Throughout the groups, we have had veterans from every branch of the military. The open studio approach and support group model open up the group to evolution and change based on the needs of the participants. The art therapist in this role serves as more of a "consultant in the art therapy journey," one who guides and helps the group to navigate discussion and different topics (Jones *et al.*, 2018, p.78).

TRUST

Trust is the foundation and the most necessary component to building any kind of healthy relationship. In therapy, trust is the crucial and anchoring base essential to creating a safe environment for clients to be able to open up to exploring, experiencing, and healing their wounds within a confidential setting (Ottemiller & Awais, 2016). Active-duty service members have minimal rights to confidential protection of information. For example, some units are not allowed to fully go on leave until everyone on the squad is physically, emotionally, and mentally able to do so. As a result, I've heard countless stories from my veteran clients of service members who came back from tours in the Middle East with layers of PTSD only to waive mental healthcare or express that they did not need counseling, so that they and members of their squad could go on leave and see their families and friends. Who could blame them? After being away from your family and friends for an extended period of time in a war zone, who would want to keep members of their unit from seeing their family and friends, let alone their own family? Veterans have disclosed that while they were serving active duty, not all records, especially mental health records, were kept confidential from their superiors, which created a strained and fractured distrust of leaders and mental health professionals trained to help soldiers.

When I entered the first veterans' group as an intern, the group members did not automatically trust me. They were inquisitive and curious watchers of my every move. It took months to build a rapport of trust. I was blessed with the opportunity to work with my first veterans' group for a whole year, which allowed ample time for the participants of the group to trust and feel safe around me. After I graduated and was no longer an intern, another intern from a different art therapy graduate program was co-leading under Jane's veterans' group for six months. She reflected that she was struggling in the group because group members did not fully trust her, noting that it took more time to build trust with veterans compared to other populations.

Group cohesiveness is considered to be the "bedrock of group experience" (Butler & Fuhriman, 1983, p.132). Cohesion informs the connection that group members experience and feel within a group and builds trust within the group. Cohesion is not built solely by the therapist, but each member has a responsibility to generate and foster cohesion within the group (Yalom, 2005). Within this cohesion, there is trust and safety, but there is also room for disagreement and more allowance of conflict (Yalom, 2005). This cohesion of trust fosters belonging and a team mindset, and opens up pathways to vulnerability. I have observed many arguments and disagreements as an intern and lead therapist in the group. Some of these arguments have ended well, encouraging healing, while others have caused further discourse, pain, and processing. One recent argument centered on politics and racism. The discussion became abruptly personal when both sides felt attacked and harsh words were exchanged. The group solution in this instance was to allow both sides to express their point of view and hurts; the group also set the boundary of not talking about politics within group sessions. One member chose to leave the group to pursue individual art therapy and work on personal goals. The group expressed that they had felt fearful at moments during the argument, almost as though the group cohesion had been broken. It took weeks of processing and reflection for the group to recover and weave together a new cohesive circle of trust.

A REFUGE OF HOPE

I have had several veterans reflect that this group was "different" from all the other groups they participated in at the VA. Some of these groups included dialectical behavior therapy groups, cognitive behavioral therapy groups, groups geared towards MST, couple's counseling groups, and prolonged exposure groups. Many group members over the years have described this art therapy support group as the "safest group" they have ever been a part of, a true refuge of hope. One observation and distinction that group members have repeatedly noticed is that the art therapy group at The Art Station has provided a safe place for exploration but also confrontation. Sadly, many group members have reflected on past groups at the VA and other veteran centers, noticing that they do not deal with the conflict in the group but rather sweep it under the rug. This feeling of safety has allowed many veterans to see hope, healing, and transformation for the first time since coming out of the military.

Yasmin (pseudonym), a 42-year-old Latina woman who served in the military for 20 years, re-entered our art therapy group after several years of taking a break. She entered quietly and tentatively, appropriately engaging with group members. Yasmin reflected that she struggled in the previous art therapy group at The Art Station because of the size and number of group members, noting that she felt "crowded." She told the group that she decided to join the morning group to have more "space" and get her out of the house during the day while her husband was at work.

Yasmin expressed that she was anxious about rejoining the group. Since Yasmin had already been through the different art mediums when she first participated in the group, I invited her to work on a simple mandala to ground her anxiety and allow her a container to express her feelings. Yasmin created her circle and then a second internal circle. She became shaky, appearing more anxious than when she started. She looked up at me saying, "I can't do this today; do you have any mandala coloring pages that I could color instead?" I brought her some mandala coloring pages. She began working on coloring in different shapes within the mandala and started to take deeper breaths, appearing visibly more relaxed and calm.

Later in the year, Yasmin chose to tackle watercolors and became extremely frustrated with the process, noticing and reflecting on her own perfectionistic tendencies and desire for her art to look a certain way. She next tried using watercolor color pencils, which provided the control she needed that day. As Yasmin continued to consistently attend the art therapy group, she became increasingly more open to sharing and being vulnerable within the group. She quickly made connections to other group members and asked thoughtful, reflective questions.

The following year, Yasmin ventured into creating acrylic pour paintings where acrylic paint and a fluid medium called Folderol are used to pour paint on canvas. She connected to the metaphor of letting go of control. She appeared soothed by the process, taking a deep breath and sharing that it felt "incredible" to "let go." Yasmin continued to grow in "letting go," choosing to try watercolors again, painting new landscapes, making an inside/outside mask, and creating more abstract art that represented her newfound freedom. She also reported getting out more socially, working out consistently, and traveling with her friends more often. Before Yasmin had started back in art therapy, she had struggled to leave the house and sometimes even get out of bed. She would often stay home and had minimal social connections outside her family. Being a part of the group and working on her personal goals increased her self-esteem and provided the impetus for her to get back out into the world. She recently had shoulder surgery, which required eight months of extensive and painful physical therapy—a much longer recovery than previous surgeries. Yasmin embraced the healing process with courage and hopefulness, acknowledging the depth of her physical pain and expressing gratitude for her past growth. She reflected on her healing, noticing that if she had experienced this slow recovery process with any of her past surgeries, she would have fallen into a "deep depression." Yasmin was also able to travel independently to a women's conference in another state by herself, reflecting, "I would not have been able to go to the conference without being a part of this group."

Recently, I shared some upcoming changes to the group dynamic. Naturally, this brought up some anxiety, so I had the group explore these feelings within individual mandalas. Yasmin thoughtfully processed her first group session, remembering how she was paralyzed with anxiety and was unable even to create a mandala, whereas now she approached the mandala with confidence, reflecting on her courage, healing, and hope as she looked to the future.

FOSTERING RESILIENCE

A resilient person is one who is able to bounce back or overcome adverse circumstances. The American Psychological Association (2014) defines resilience as "the process of adapting well in the face of adversity, trauma, tragedy, threats or even significant sources of stress (para. 4)." Andi (pseudonym), a young African American female, joined the group at the end of my internship. She would often join in with discussions, sharing stories from her experiences in Iraq and Afghanistan, appearing to relate to peers with similar experiences. Andi attended the group almost every other week. When Andi started feeling more comfortable in the group, she opened up one-on-one to me about a stalker who had followed her from another group at another clinic and had found an assortment of extensive and creative ways to stalk her by trying to access her through social media, using fake accounts. She reflected further that this unwelcome person had discovered her new phone number, even after she had changed it. As Andi continued to attend the group, she continued to express frustration and anger towards her unwelcome stalker. Andi shared that she had considered getting a restraining order. She appeared more relieved after each group when she was able to express her internal stress and feelings of harassment through words and art. Other group members would express empathy and encourage Andi, showing support and offering ideas for protection. She was often focused on drawing as a way of coping with anxiety and intrusive thoughts.

When the time came for the group to add more group members,

Andi was asked if she wanted to share the name of her stalker, who was also a veteran. She chose not to and, as a result, her stalker found her and entered the group. The results of this interchange were disastrous and volatile with Andi slamming an easel down on the ground and yelling, "Get away from me! Stop following me!" Andi's stalker was escorted out of the room, debriefed, and referred elsewhere. Andi was still struggling to catch up with her adrenaline when I rejoined the group. She expressed anger, resentment towards her stalker, and hatred. She practiced taking deep breaths. Andi returned the following week and consistently attended every week for months. During this time, Andi verbally processed her emotions and frustrations towards her stalker and created art that calmed and grounded her to the present (see Figure 4.1). Over time, Andi's anxiety related to her stalker lowered as she had a safe place to recover and heal even after experiencing such an explosive moment within the same space. Andi's resilience grew brilliantly as she refused to let the incident with her stalker keep her from attending the one group in which she felt safe.

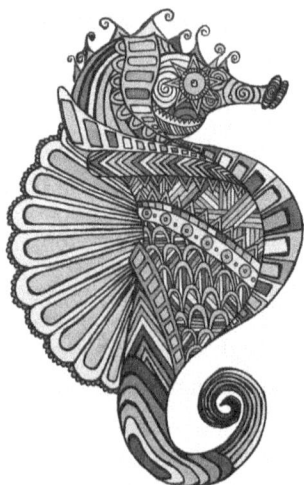

Figure 4.1: Andi's art

A SENSE OF SELF

Bill (pseudonym), a Caucasian male in his 50s, entered the support group while I was still an intern. He shared that he had never taken an art class. He expressed feeling insecure and intimidated. Bill explored all of the different mediums presented through the introductory open studio model and decided to focus his full attention on drawing. Bill consistently arrived early to the group to work on his sketches, often taking a taxi or riding his bike because he had never got his driver's license. He also purchased his own art materials that he brought each week. Early on in the group, he displayed a quiet demeanor. He sat away from peers, often appearing private and guarded. Bill would frequently join in the group conversation by sharing his opinion about certain military situations and his knowledge about movies and musicals. One day, Bill arrived late to the group with blood on his face and wearing his cycling attire. With wide eyes and adrenaline pumping, he explained that he had been in an accident where a car had cut him off when he was trying to cross the street, which caused him to flip off his bike. This traumatic event did not deter or prevent Bill from attending the group. He went to the VA to attend to his medical needs and returned to the group the following week by way of taxi.

Bill began to express to me in the group that he was wanting to express more of his feminine side through art and eventually start taking ballet classes, reflecting that he had been chastised as a child for requesting to take ballet classes. Bill reflected that he was afraid of his father's rejection and castigation. The subject of Bill's drawings originally displayed more masculine components of landscapes and comics, with one specific drawing of "War of the Worlds" from the original comic. Bill reflected that as a child he was absorbed in the vast arena of comics. After finishing his "War of the Worlds" drawing, he shared his experience of seeing a fellow soldier, who was only four feet away from him, explode from an improvised explosive device (IED) (see Figure 4.2). He tearfully reflected that he did not know why he had been spared and allowed to live, while his fellow soldier's life had ended so abruptly. After this drawing was completed, Bill chose to draw mermaids, fashion models, and creative perspective drawings of Disney princesses (see Figure 4.3). It was almost as if the "War of the Worlds" drawing represented a part of his past self, upbringing, and military experiences, whereas the more feminine drawings symbolized his embrace of a new chapter of his life. Bill started taking ballet classes every week with group and individual lessons. He expressed that he felt more like himself than ever in his life. Through the art therapy process, Bill was able to explore a side of himself that he was not allowed to express as a child or while in the military.

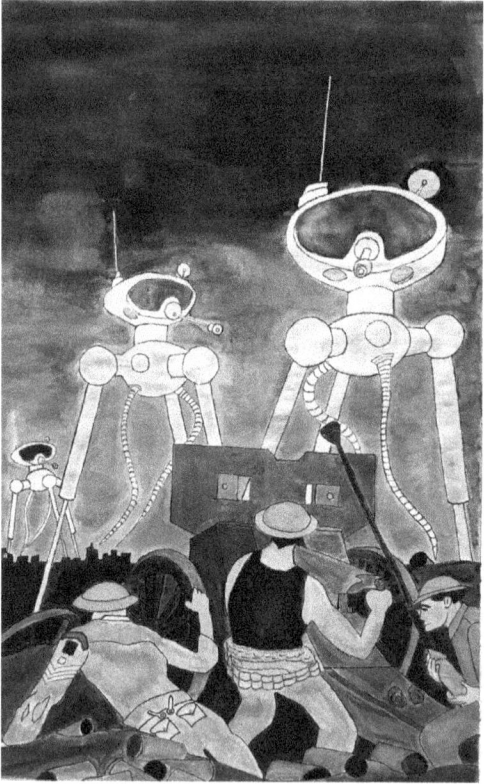

Figure 4.2: Bill's "War of the Worlds" drawing

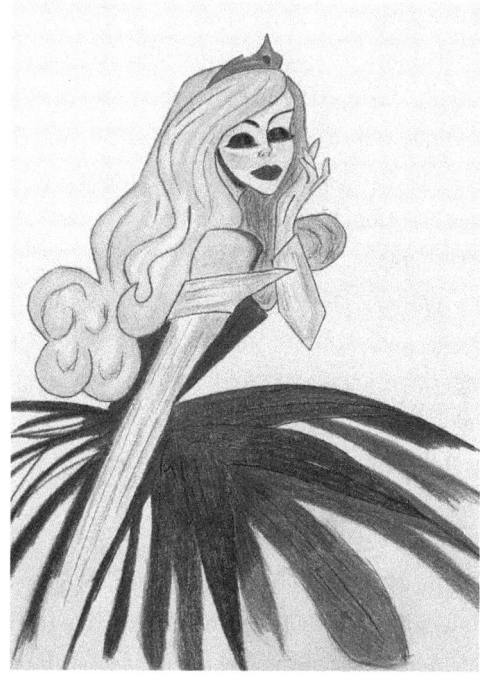

Figure 4.3: A drawing made by Bill after his "War of the Worlds" drawing

As Bill embraced this new chapter of expression, he reflected on his military experiences, noticing that he missed the structure of the military but not the lack of individuality. Bill often expressed that it felt as if he was able to make choices now for things he was truly passionate and interested in after his growth within the art therapy group. Bill's confidence and passion for his art increased as he began to add mediums such as acrylic and watercolor paint to his drawings. He showed his artwork at fundraisers and art shows displaying veterans' art. Bill also began working on his drawings while at a bar, or in restaurants, proudly sharing his artwork with those who would ask about it.

CATHARTIC BREAKTHROUGHS

Traumatic experiences are often stored in the non-verbal portion of the brain (van der Kolk, 2014). When trauma occurs in people, the Broca's area (responsible for producing language) of the brain shuts down, and the amygdala takes over and captures the details of the traumatic experience visually through bodily sensation (Rausch *et al.*, 1996). Art therapy has a unique way of processing traumatic memories by utilizing sensory output. Lusebrink's (2004) research showed that engaging the senses activates emotional responses in the amygdala. Lobban (2014) also stated: "Art therapy is an action therapy that combines movement, tactility, vision, memory, and imagery in the creative process and which addresses the non-verbal core of traumatic memories" (p.11).

Betty (pseudonym), a 40-year-old Caucasian woman, had been in and out of the art therapy group for ten years, experiencing the art therapy group at the VA, and the University of Texas at Arlington, and at The Art Station. She had been involved in extracurricular activities and gone back to school in different seasons of a ten-year period. When she reconnected to the group, her vivacious personality immediately shone through her interactions with group members as she rekindled friendships and made new connections. Betty started off with her "doodling," which comprised a meditative process of creating maze-like drawings of lines that zigzagged throughout different corners of her paper. She reflected that the process was calming and centering as she breathed more deeply and allowed the art to take over the direction. She also noted that she had been using this drawing process throughout her life to help her cope with the trauma and abuse around her. Betty described her childhood as "challenging," often reflecting on her painful upbringing and familial dysfunction. Her parents divorced when she was young, which further exasperated already present emotional divisions between her and her siblings. She expressed a deep desire to be close to her siblings as adults and form a tight-knit connection.

As Betty took art classes at a local university, she noticed that her freedom of expression and creativity were not always honored or respected, often reflecting on the specific confining expectations of one of her art professors. She continued to create her maze-like drawings for anxiety relief, often expressing a desire for deeper connection in her friendships and acquaintances. As her drawings evolved, she noticed characters or people within her drawings, observing similarities between her artwork and the artist Keith Haring. At one point during the group, she contained the zigzag lines within a mandala on black Artagain paper, highlighting their line value and dancing trails of color (see Figure 4.4). Betty reflected that the lines represented different paths and avenues of choices that had led her to her current journey of healing. Her artwork often reflected deep themes of loss, such as loss of her parents, loss of connection with family, loss of a friendship due to suicide, leaving high school before graduation, and loss of trust in men due to sexual abuse.

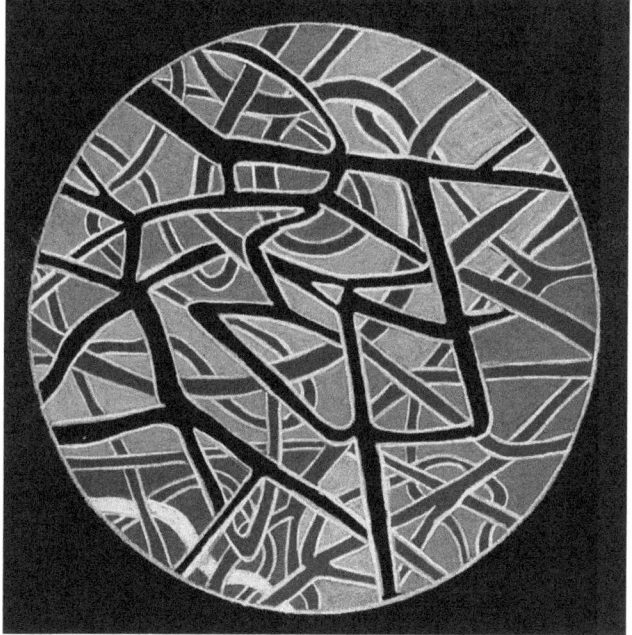

Figure 4.4: Betty's mandala

While processing past trauma, Betty created a "May Day" timeline, highlighting traumatic events that occurred in the past during the month of May. She reflected on the depth of her pain as she tearfully recounted the impact of the trauma. She expressed her pain by using colorful flowers to represent somber events. She described the process as "freeing" in helping her surrender the past and embrace the present.

Betty acknowledged that it was not fully up to her to reconcile and rebuild connections with her siblings. She was able to take ownership of her part of the relationship and surrender her expectations as to how her siblings should respond to her desire for connection.

One day, Betty entered the open studio tearfully expressing wounds of sorrow, noticing how her past trauma of emotional abuse within her family was affecting her in the present. This particular day, Betty was the only group member able to make it to the session. As she sat down, I checked in with her and asked her what she needed during this time. As streams of tears slid down her face, she responded by saying, "I need to get these feelings out!" Betty acknowledged her emotions of sadness, fear, shame, embarrassment, frustration, and anger. She first wrote them down and gave them a voice. Tactile media evokes an emotional response and aids in the expression of emotions (Lusebrink, 2004). So, we used clay throwing to engage the kinesthetic and sensory attributes of the medium to communicate and dispel her trapped emotions. Betty's tears began to subside as she energetically threw the clay down and was able to give a voice to her emotions. She described herself as feeling "empowered" to be able to express and challenge her emotions instead of containing them within her body. Betty acknowledged that she felt "lighter" from the cathartic release, noticing that the physical pain in her shoulders and her stomach pain had dissipated. "Once the deleterious effects of the traumatic event have been reversed then one can proceed to working on the meaning of the event, but not before. This is a reversal of the usual sequence of therapy" (Gantt & Tinnin, 2009, p.151). Once Betty was able to process the pain directly related to the trauma, such as the physical pain in her shoulders and stomach, she was able to delve more deeply into the meaning of the events.

COURAGEOUS METAMORPHOSIS

The Art Station recently received a new grant for the veterans' art therapy support group. Future changes and additions to the group were communicated to the group. The existing group members have a combined 15 years' experience of being in the group. Change is always hard, and exceptionally hard after experiencing powerful, healing breakthroughs with group members. These group members have spent months—even years—being in the trenches of expressing personal stories of trauma and overcoming fears. The group acknowledged their trepidation, frustration, and sadness with the future changes. Group members channeled their emotions into their artwork, reflecting on their individual growth within the group. Some members reflected on their emotional bravery in stepping out of their comfort zone to show up to the group and to trust the process. Another member reflected on her resilience in overcoming and healing from past trauma, acknowledging how the group art therapy process had increased her confidence and ability to overcome setbacks and barriers. One veteran reflected on how the future change could be a greater avenue for displaying growth.

Two weeks later, another grant was offered to provide an opportunity for community partnership between The Art Station and a glass studio in the area. The grant outlined a partnership that utilized a glass-building instructor along with an art therapist. The grant stipulated that the two veterans' art therapy groups at the Art Station would merge together into one group. Both groups agreed to this change and expressed both excitement and anxiety about trying something new. The group agreed that this new transition could be a positive step towards growing their confidence in using a new medium, and would provide opportunities to get out in the community in a new way. This new group successfully started in the fall of 2019 but was unfortunately disbanded due to Covid-19 restrictions.

While waiting for this new group and partnership to commence, the group requested a closure directive to process their growth. Group members described how art therapy had transformed their everyday lives of seclusion, avoidance, and withdrawal from society into an active presence of engaging within their communities through social groups, art classes, exercising at gyms, and taking courses at university. For the art directive, the group was asked to paint a butterfly using a watercolor resist process. The resistive components of using a white crayon represented the struggle and empowerment in overcoming fears and breaking through barriers. The watercolor colors symbolized their personal growth process. One group member used the white crayon to draw a symmetrical pattern that represented her consistency in attending the group even when it was hard. As she painted over the white crayon she felt as though she had made a mistake but was quickly reminded by the group that there are "no mistakes in art therapy." She used this "mistake" to remind herself of her "steadiness" and resilience to rise above her anxiety and depression and not give up.

Another group member divided her butterfly into two sections. One section represented how she came into the group, while the other side symbolized her growth. One side was labeled "fear" with dark colors of red, black, brown, and purple, and the other side was titled "free" with lighter, pastel colors of yellow, green, blue, and orange. She described herself as entering the group with "extreme social anxiety" and fear of sharing. Her freedom side spoke to her new-found metamorphosis of independence and confidence to face her fears and overcome a decade of social withdrawal. Another group member did not fully finish painting her butterfly, describing it as "representational" that her healing journey was not finished yet (see Figure 4.5). She reflected on the challenges of change and powerfully reiterated a quote she had previously used in the group: "It's not life-ending, it is life-changing." The metamorphosis of courage shone through the life changes of each individual.

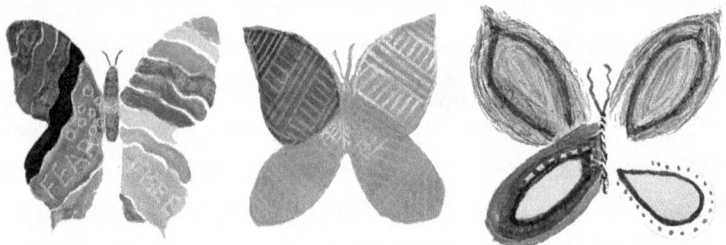

Figure 4.5: Butterfly images created by group members

CONCLUSIONS

Military service members who come out of the military need a safe place to rediscover themselves, to heal from the brokenness of their world and the trauma they have observed and experienced, to learn new ways of coping in an ever-changing world, and where they feel safe and can trust those around them. The systems and programs in our world put in place for active service members returning from multiple military duties have often been bereft of providing holistic care to meet the versatile needs of veterans.

The veterans I have had the privilege of working with described a greater need for groups that establish a firm foundation of trust and safety. Group members, especially the female veterans in my group, often described that they did not know whom they could trust while serving in the military. These women often banded together with other women service members, acknowledging that there was safety in numbers. Group members described a need for therapy groups that were not afraid to confront group members who were rude, disrespectful, and disruptive to the group. This art therapy group has been a refreshing respite and refuge for healing and breakthroughs in confronting personal fears and external conflict within a safe environment centered on trust. Within the layers of trust, group cohesion was found to be essential for vulnerability to blossom.

Resilience in overcoming fears and personal barriers to goals was encouraged through the group art therapy process. New connections to past experiences were created and seen from fresh perspectives and angles. The group provided a safe container for expression, encouragement, and support. Fostering resilience created insight into increasing and developing personal coping skills for anxiety and depression. Art therapy provided an avenue to expel negative thoughts, a distraction from intrusive thoughts, and a place to rebuild and restore broken dreams. A sense of self and individuality was established through the art process and exploration of materials. Often service members do not have the opportunity to engage in personal self-care activities and life-enriching activities. Life in the military is often focused on the bigger picture, the group, not the individual needs of each service member. The art materials provided a playful stage to trust the process and not rely so heavily on the end product. This art therapy group provided an opportunity for group members to traverse through their own uncharted territory of discovering and re-discovering their personal preferences, opinions, and viewpoints.

Cathartic breakthroughs eventuated through the group art therapy process when veterans processed past trauma using sensory oriented mediums such as clay and watercolor. The sensory stimulus of the materials provided an outlet for acutely buried trauma to surface after layers of past experiences had been safely processed and expelled. The cathartic dispelling of negative emotions afforded room for positive emotions and memories to take root. The open studio approach to art therapy provided an adaptable opportunity of choice to process loss in whatever medium was most helpful and applicable to their experience. These opportunities for choice and flexibility empowered veterans with the space to reframe their experiences in their own way and in their own time. Group art therapy creates a safe place for "intense affects" to be contained and explored "safely without retribution" (Thompson, 2009, p.164).

Just as a butterfly emerges after an intake of nutrients, transitional rest, body transformation, and strengthening of its muscle by escaping the confines of the chrysalis, the veterans in this group transformed their fears into courage by taking in encouragement and positivity from the group, making time for rest and play, and visually breaking through their past constraints; morphing them into a freedom of flight through the art therapy process. This freedom of flight created a steadiness and willingness to attend group and fight together against the darkest of nights to overcome social anxiety and withdrawal. As the group members shared their courageous metamorphosis through their butterfly paintings, they reminded each other of past hindrances that no longer obstructed their growth. They reflected on the art process and the challenge of seeing that "there are no mistakes in art therapy, just new directions," admiring their strength to overcome setbacks related to stalkers, past trauma, group disruptions, and broken relationships.

Chapter 5

Reflection, Reminiscence, Honor: Working with Veterans in Later Life

—— ERIN PARTRIDGE ——

Aging veterans may choose or need to live in assisted living settings in their later life. These places may be civilian or specialized care provided as a benefit to those who served. Assisted living and memory care settings can simultaneously be places of confirmation and erasure for older adult veterans. Many communities honor and celebrate service members on holidays and invite story sharing and reminiscence. These same communities, because of the perpetuation of outdated models of group offerings and social engagement (Partridge, 2019a), may discourage or silence older veterans when they attempt to discuss painful experiences, work through strong feelings, or process unresolved trauma related to service. Art therapists working in older adult settings offer a supportive space for reflection that spans the whole continuum of human emotion.

TRAUMA AND REMINISCENCE

Recent efforts to support active-duty and recently returned veterans is a positive step in the holistic wellbeing of service members (Berberian, Walker & Kaimal, 2018; Kaimal *et al.*, 2018; Lobban, 2016). Many of those who served in the conflicts of decades past have not had access to this wider range of services, and may not have a formal diagnosis (Davison *et al.*, 2016). Returning service members from World War II, especially those with visible wounds or amputations, "carried collective and national anxieties about the transition from wartime to civilian labor and its relation to the precarious status of the male body" (Serlin, 2006, p.50). The research and clinical literature suggest that even for those who have worked through trauma related to military service, the aging process prompts a need for renewed support and processing: "In later life many combat Veterans confront and rework their wartime memories in an effort to find meaning and build coherence" (Davison *et al.*, 2016, p. 14), a process the authors labeled "later-adulthood trauma reengagement." For older veterans, their service in the military may have included combat as well as more positive experiences such as education or vocational training. Veterans benefit from opportunities to explore these seemingly opposing categories of experience in order to resolve confusion and come to terms with ambivalence about their service. Depending on when they served, they may currently receive honor and respect for their service, or they may be faced with stereotyping and disdain. For example, veterans returning from Vietnam faced complicated situations as they re-entered civilian life; their deployment during young adulthood and the negative public opinion about the war had far-reaching implications for their employment and long-term wellbeing (National Advisory Council on Vocational Education, 1972). Their experiences did not include as many opportunities for processing and working through their service:

> Because of the fierce opposition to the war and the polarizing debates that tore apart the nation, many of the veterans who returned home felt they were wearing a shroud of shame for their participation in an unpopular war. Guilt-ridden about their experiences, the veterans were often unable or unwilling to share their experiences with relatives, friends, or coworkers. They paid a heavy price for their involvement in Vietnam and for decades of silence. (Berman, 2015, p.515)

As they age, this silence can stimulate negative or maladaptive behaviors, depression, or increased feelings of isolation. Therapists working with this group of unseen or stigmatized veterans need to address the shame and guilt as part of the treatment goals. Art therapists working with veterans in residential or medical settings need to look and listen for manifestations of guilt, shame, and other maladaptive behavior in the art and art therapy sessions, as they may manifest in different ways from those we see in civilian populations.

When working in older adult settings, the type of reminiscence matters. Studies show that reminiscing to assuage boredom, one of the self-negative forms of reminiscence, can cast the current moment in a negative view and exacerbate depression (Cappeliez, 2019). Boredom reminiscence is a particular danger for people living in assisted living; many traditional forms of programming rely heavily on recitation of facts or trivia (Partridge, 2019a) and can unintentionally prime residents to engage in recitation of life stories out of boredom. For older adult veterans, who may have traveled, fought, and explored as part of their active duty, older adult care contexts understandably seem dull by comparison. Reminiscence needs to be guided: "Simply encouraging older depressed individuals to recollect personal memories may have the very adverse effect of activating a downward spiral, unless they are provided with the guiding context to review these memories" (Cappeliez, 2019, p.241). Introducing reminiscence needs to include careful planning and knowledge of the client. The therapist should be ready to explore traumatic experiences and guide reminiscence for productive, healthy outcomes. Art therapists working with imagery, art process, and language have several channels through which to guide reminiscence and reflection, giving these professionals a potential advantage in addressing the needs of aging veterans. By gently redirecting repetitive boredom reminiscence through the introduction of art materials and directives designed to stimulate new forms of reminiscence, the art therapist helps shift the client towards more productive and enriching ways to engage in story sharing.

QUIET ACKNOWLEDGEMENT

Personal, historical, and social context matters. Photos of older adult veterans in their uniforms around assisted living buildings can be interpreted as deeply respectful or trite, depending on how they are contextualized. If these photos only come out on significant holidays, we miss the possibility for therapeutic and growth-oriented work. Instead, we should create opportunities for creating a rich context for these photos. Likewise, the common practice of posting pictures of the veteran's uniformed younger selves on their door in assisted living means we miss the human currently before us and see them only through their youth. Uniformed portraits and photos from service offer an opportunity for older adults, family members, and the art therapist to create places of visual acknowledgement and honor for the veteran. Similar to the memorial process described as part of work with families (Partridge, 2019a), the art therapist can support creating visual art that incorporates photos from a veteran's time in service. These can be ornate, multimedia pieces or simple frames. Involving multiple generations in this process creates an opportunity for older adults to share stories and impart wisdom. As a group process in assisted living or memory care settings, it can bring veterans together around their shared experiences—things they may not discuss with their civilian neighbors. These projects also allow for varied levels of verbal discussion—where silence is a "legitimate choice" (Reda, 2009, p.6) people can make. We need to respect the aging veterans' need to not talk. Creating a frame or adding one's own photo to a community celebration might be the right level of acknowledgement for some veterans—therapists should guard against making assumptions about this silence.

Gerald, a resident in assisted living who was generally very quiet about his service, came downstairs for breakfast with a wrinkled, black and white photograph of himself propped up against a milk carton on his walker. He had turned the photo to face forward, so that people approaching him could see it. The photo showed him at age 20 in his dress uniform; with broad shoulders and a bright smile he faced the camera looking invincible. On closer inspection, as he made his way into the dining room, I noticed he also had his army hat tucked into a pocket of his sweatpants that day. His display was getting the desired reaction—people were stopping him to comment on how handsome he looked; remarks to which he responded with a big grin. It was the first time I had seen him smile in a long time. Gerald was experiencing increased distress from Parkinson's disease—his symptoms had worsened and he was no longer able to be as independent as he wanted. His gait and posture prompted the care team to restrict his trips out in the community on his own. His limited mobility also restricted his clothing choices; the symptoms of Parkinson's necessitated oversized soft cotton shirts and sweatpants, things he could easily pull on and off without buttons or other fasteners. His new uniform was far different from the dress uniform in the photo. Creating a makeshift display of a photo of himself from a vital stage of his life communicated his need to be seen as strong, independent, and able. He used the photo to communicate who he was before the Parkinson's.

Seeing his crumpled photo on its makeshift frame, at risk for more wrinkles and spilled milk, prompted me to invite him to join us in the art studio after lunch to create a frame for his photo. He agreed to come, despite never joining us before. First, I asked him to use a ruler to measure a rectangle one inch larger than his photograph on all sides and draw it out on a piece of heavy bookboard. Though cardboard will work, bookboard is thicker and more substantial—communicating to the veteran that you value what they are working on. While he worked on that task, I made a color photocopy of his photo; when possible, working with high-quality photocopies reduces the risk of damage to these precious memorabilia. We can also photocopy other important items like medals or name badges for inclusion. When I returned with the copies, he asked for assistance in cutting the bookboard. His request was such a positive sign—because I started the session by giving him a task and encouraging him to work independently, he felt safe enough to ask for assistance later. A boost in self-esteem from all the compliments he received that day also supported his ability to ask for help. Once we had it cut, we were ready to wrap his frame. Working with a sheet of thin copper, we covered the bookboard rectangle. Slowly and methodically, he folded the edges of the copper over the back of the board. He experimented with creating patterns on a scrap piece of copper, but decided he liked the clean lines of the plain copper frame. We cut out and glued the copy of the photo down onto the copper and he held it up for everyone to admire.

For the next few months, that photo had a place of honor on his walker or on the windowsill in his room. The process of working with his photo did not necessitate much verbal exchange about his service or his current experience. He seemed to need the quiet acknowledgement of tending to the photo of himself and thereby that part of himself. Though it could have been an opening into overt discussion of his past or of his feelings about the symptoms of Parkinson's, it did not feel therapeutically necessary. As with recent research on the impact of clay manipulation for people living with Parkinson's (Elkis-Abuhoff & Gaydos, 2018), creating the frame for his image was a kinesthetic process with potential somatic benefits along with the emotional benefits. With aging veterans, we need to balance where we dive deeper into their emotional experiences and where we stay in the metaphor with the art process. For Gerald, tending to his sense of self was the most sensitive and ethical course of action. He needed time to navigate between independence and need for assistance on his own terms as he engaged in the cognitive task of measurement and tactile task of bending the copper. The positive experience in the session also created an opening for him to return to the studio in the last years of his life—he came several other times to talk and sit with us.

SUDDEN DISCLOSURES

The need for reminiscence and later-life trauma re-engagement (Davison *et al.*, 2016) can result in sudden or unexpected disclosures of trauma or difficult combat-related experiences. In these instances, the art therapist needs to provide a safe and open environment for older adult veterans to explore and express what comes up. Depending on the setting, this may involve being prepared to set limits about what is discussed when—keeping the service member and their peers emotionally safe. Particularly in assisted living and memory care, where people may have difficulty separating past historical events from current circumstances, we need to be sure that one person's need for reminiscence is not upsetting or frightening to a peer.

One veteran I interacted with would start spilling his story almost before we said our hellos; he started talking as soon as I sat down at the table where he was working on some coloring pages set out by a staff member in the assisted living building. His speech, pressured and emotionally charged, covered topics one does not usually dive into with strangers. As I sat and listened, it seemed as if he just really needed to tell his story to someone. He veered wildly from topic to topic—talking about the bird images he was coloring, his travel and military service, his business experiences, and his family. Each time I spoke, he made a pun or other play on the words I used. It became clear that the puns were both a way to connect and a way to take control of our interaction—to signal to me that he was the one who needed to talk. The therapist can introduce silence into the session to "demonstrate empathy and give the client time to feel or think" (Regev, Kurt & Snir, 2016, p.86). Sometimes our role with aging veterans is to be a trusted, active listener. We may need to stay silent longer to allow for the longer processing time of aging clients (Gosselin & Gagné, 2011; Pike, 2013). I found that the more quiet and attentive I was as we sat and colored together, his speech slowed down and we entered into a more relaxed conversational cadence.

Another veteran, Thomas, never attended the open studio art therapy groups in the assisted living community where he lived. With staff prompting, he began to come to social events, but he rarely discussed his life or experiences. The one glimpse into his life prior to assisted living came in the form of dance—his eyes lit up when music played and he would leap to his feet and find a dance partner. We knew his veteran status because of family disclosure and his favorite accessory: his Navy hat.

He had never shown an interest in art or in attending our groups, so it was a surprise when he sat down with me one day during in informal art group on the floor where he lived. He sat up tall in his chair wearing his Navy hat, watching quietly as I distributed projects and supplies to some of his peers. When I turned to greet him, he tapped the brim of his hat and asked if I liked it. Before I could answer, he noticed a blue marker and his eyes welled up with tears. His tears surprised me, as I had never seen him emote so much. I acknowledged his emotion aloud: "It seems as if you're experiencing some strong emotions right now; do you want to tell me about what you're feeling?" He reached out and picked up the blue marker and held it up at eye level very close to his face. Then he set it down, made eye contact with me, and said "I forgot about *that* blue." I asked him to tell me more about what "*that* blue" meant to him. He took a deep breath and told me about the blue skies he saw through the windows of the fighter planes he flew in. He took his hat off and placed it on the table in front of him, tapping it periodically as he continued to talk. He was speaking more than I had ever heard before—he usually interacted via short sentences or single words. His gaze was out beyond me or anyone at the table and his voice sounded far away. He told us about how it seemed so strange that they were "up there to shoot" but seeing so much beauty in the skies. His words described what many veterans experience—the sometimes jarring contrast between beauty and pain, exhilaration and fear, camaraderie and human suffering.

I asked him if he would like to try making some marks with that blue color to make a picture. He picked up the marker again, but hesitated to remove the cap or make any marks. After sitting with him for a few more minutes, I suggested we trace his hand on the page so he could have a place to start. I carefully traced around his hand and we joked when we noticed the marker leaked and we both had ink on our fingers. Once he saw his hand on the page, he was able to start making long arcing strokes with the marker across the top of the page. His marks looked like the earth's curvature—something I noticed, but did not speak aloud. He continued to make curving blue lines for a while longer. Then he set the marker down, sighed deeply, and looked out the window: "I can't get over that blue," he said quietly. I asked him if he had anything else he wanted to share about the color or about his art. He paused, tilted the art up to face himself, and then asked if he could put it up in his room. He said he did not ever want to forget *that* blue.

The interaction with him was brief but impactful. The color and mark-making enabled us to have a conversation about what he had experienced and created space for him to express aloud some fears about lost memories. His simple image was a record of this very honest, personal disclosure—sharing an unexpected memory with the group.

SERVICE MEMBERS IN A CIVILIAN MILIEU

Some of the shorthand that permeates assisted living settings can pigeon-hole veterans in a single aspect of their life. Residents and staff lapse into referring to people by their previous occupation or some other notable fact. Particularly at move-in, a person's veteran status can shape how we think about them. Staff may decorate the person's door with imagery related to their service or address them inappropriately with salutes or incorrect honorifics. We need to set the example with staff to proceed carefully; we do not know all the details of someone's service history. Letting the older adults dictate how they want to be addressed and what of their history they want to share is important.

Camille's experience moving into assisted living offers a good example of this pigeon-holing. She attended a social event on her first afternoon in the building. One staff member, having learned she worked as a code breaker during World War II introduced her as "our code breaker" and then proceeded to ask a lot of specific questions about her work. This woman nervously laughed and repeated, "I'm just Camille" over and over—trying to claim her current identity rather than her former occupation. Gently steering the conversation towards her current interests helped her relax and get to know her peers. It also relieved her of the need to be the community's history teacher.

One example of a veteran whose life cannot be defined by his service history alone was Mario. He served in Vietnam in the Air Force.

When he returned to the United States, he studied psychology and became interested in human behavior on the community and societal level—his interests eventually led him to become a vociferous anti-nuclear proliferation protestor and he was incarcerated several times as a result of his activism. When he moved into assisted living, his veteran status only came up in conversations when he was coordinating his medical appointments at the local VA hospital. He was much better known as an activist, especially after his arrest at a protest during his time as a resident in assisted living; the arresting officer cuffed him improperly (behind his back) given his age and use of a mobility aid. His near-fall caused a big uproar in the local media. His dual identity as a veteran and a protestor enabled a very interesting conversation between him and an internment camp survivor. After watching a documentary about World War II, the two of them lingered and talked about the unexpected commonalities they shared. They discussed their experiences of incarceration and their attitudes about war now in their later lives. The woman who experienced internment told Mario about one soldier who was friendly and her inability to see him that way until recently. Mario shared that his ongoing activism was a direct result of what he saw and experienced in combat. They both felt their experiences made them more effective activists and they connected via both of their efforts to build community.

EVOLVING MEMORY

As service members age and experience later life, their access to their memories may be less clear. We need to make space for reminiscence and reflection in the art—without needing them to "stick to the facts." The complicated, overlapping collective and personal histories of conflict, military service, and individual lives get even more complicated when service members experience dementia. Some of Camille's discomfort about being labeled a code breaker may have been about fears that she could not live up to the label with the correct stories. All our life stories connect to our cultures; "Cultures define the shape of a life" (Fivush &

Booker, 2019, p.111), especially the lives of those who define our culture on the world stage. Unlike most personal or professional stories, the stories of aging veterans are tied closely to historical facts. There can be an impulse to draw direct lines between an individual's personal experience and written history texts.

Veterans experience different levels of later-life distress depending on their status. In a study of decorated versus non-decorated veterans, researchers looked at their psychiatric distress, imposterism, and isolation (Stein *et al.*, 2019). The researchers measured combat exposure and psychiatric distress in the veteran's middle age, and psychiatric distress, negative life events, imposterism, and isolation in their later life. They found that decorated veterans had less psychiatric distress in both middle and later life, a finding they hypothesized may be due to experiencing less imposterism and loneliness than non-decorated veterans. They emphasized the need for more research on the psychosocial aspects of aging veterans—this recommendation connects to the larger call to address loneliness and isolation in the older adult population (Wilson & Moulton, 2010). It also supports creating enrichment programs focused on the whole person rather than on one aspect of their history—particularly in settings where the majority of the population are civilians.

When I first met Frank in the memory care community, he rolled up his sleeves to show me his tattoos and asked if I had any to show him. I turned the conversation back to his tattoos, asking when he got them and what they meant to him. He touched each one in turn, telling me about the different ports he visited during his time in the Navy. He laughed, remembering a friend who was afraid to get any tattoos: "I got enough for both of us!" Frank was a slight but strong man who had a habit of pacing the memory care floor, testing exits and attempting to leave through the locked doors with visitors or staff. In staff meetings about his behavior when he first moved in, he was described as agitated; however, understanding the full context of the floor explained the pacing and door testing. When he moved into the community, he had a higher level of verbal, physical, and cognitive functioning than any of his peers, whose dementia was far more advanced. Frank's move was precipitated by increased wandering; he wandered long distances enabled by his bodily strength. He got lost in his city for hours at a time and his family wanted to keep him safe. He needed some individualized social engagement, because the rest of the people living in memory care at that time benefited from more sensory-based work and the groups were not interesting to Frank. I saw him for individual art therapy for several months, offering him undivided attention and space to talk. He readily engaged in art making, despite wondering aloud if it was "girly stuff," a common misconception in older adult settings (Partridge, 2019b). Our sessions incorporated both directive and open topic foci, depending on how he presented when I arrived to meet with him. Sometimes he was smiling and waiting for me and other times I had to seek him out in the far corners of the floor, usually testing the exit doors or sitting dejected, having failed to find a way out.

We met for our sessions in a quiet part of memory care, away from the main activity room. I noticed he was easily distracted if he could hear people in the activity room, but once we were at our "spot" he was able to focus and remain present for one or two hours. Each time we met, I brought paper, watercolors, oil pastels, and markers. Occasionally he asked for a pencil, but most of the time he was able to jump right into creating with color. If he had a hard time starting, I suggested adding a border to his page or gave him a prompt; however, most sessions he wanted to talk and create about topics of his choosing.

One day, unprompted, he started to tell part of his story: "It was like bathwater," he said, after filling the lower half of a page with blues and greens. "Is that strange to say? It is the truth though! I never expected the water to be so warm." After asking a few clarifying questions, I realized he was talking about a ship he was on during the war. They were struck by torpedoes and had to jump into the water to get to lifeboats. As he continued to paint and talk about the experience, his voice shook and he started to cry. He told me he felt guilty that he remembered the temperature of the water and exactly how it felt, but could not remember the names of those who did not survive that day. We talked about how strange memory can be and how sometimes we remember with our senses better than with our words. Work with Frank was well served by the open nature of our art sessions. He could engage in the story of his experience without needing to have all the facts exactly right. The multi-sensory art process stimulated narrative more reliant on the senses than on sequential facts. He was able to express both his lived experience as well as his present-moment guilt about lost memories, perhaps enabling him to enter into a larger conversation about memory loss and dementia.

THE ART THERAPISTS' ROLE

Art therapists working with service members in older adult settings need to be careful not to tokenize the service of veteran residents. Their service histories are not convenient programming or opportunities for historical trivia. The work we do with older adult veterans can support their self-esteem and thereby reduce their susceptibility to loneliness (Zhao, Zhang & Ran, 2017). We need to monitor discussions in mixed groups of residents, listening for situations where the probing questions of civilians may trigger trauma responses or shame about fading memories. We also need to be wary of the potential to put service members on high pedestals, leaving them with no outlet for their evolving or ambivalent feelings about their experiences. Art therapy can introduce opportunities for aging service members to reflect on their experiences at the micro and macro level: their unique memories like "*that* blue" and the bath water ocean, as well as participation in larger sociocultural dialogue through activism.

Art therapists can also assist service members to find a sense of purpose through art processes. For an aging Navy veteran with severe diabetes and limited mobility, finding a project he could do to serve his new community was very beneficial (Partridge, 2019b). This resident did not want to join the open studio group or come to the art studio, partially because of a perceived stigma about therapy and partially because his mobility was very limited. He showed me some knotted keychains he had created and asked for my assistance in procuring materials. He originally wanted to create them for staff, but his eyes lit up when he heard the suggestion of making them for residents living on the memory care floor. I told him about how distressing it was to some that they no longer had any keys when they moved into memory care and he wondered aloud if the keychain might help with the distress they expressed when reaching into their pockets and coming up empty. I gave him a list of first initials of each memory care resident and he got to work. Presenting those keychains to the residents in memory care was one of his last acts of service before he died. Though it may have seemed like a small act, it meant a great deal to this proud man with so much of his self-worth and identity attached to being of service to others. Interactions supporting the creation and gift of crafted items falls outside the normal scope of work art therapists learn about and expect to encounter, but the most important thing is to meet the client where they are. This service member needed to feel a sense of purpose, and he found it by creating for others in ways he may not have had in the open studio or a formal art therapy group.

When working with service members with dementia, we need to maintain awareness of the evolving narrative as the disease progresses. Their "narrative may become non-verbal, yet is still rich with imagery and imbued with meaning, giving a thick, rich description of a life lived" (Bryden, 2019, p.218). This phenomenon can be observed in aging service members and makes art therapy an especially appropriate choice for formal and informal treatment. Art therapy is a way to dwell in the place where the service member's need for narrative and reminiscence overlaps with their changing cognitive status; it shifts and evolves as they age to support their holistic wellbeing.

Chapter 6

Moral Injury in Veterans and Military Service Members

— RACHEL MIMS —

Moral injury (MI) is a relatively new topic in the literature. It is not a diagnosable condition but it is experienced by many veterans and it can have a huge impact on their lives. For example, Purcell *et al.* (2016) found MI impacted spirituality, sense of self, and relationships with others, and often resulted in feelings of guilt or shame. This chapter provides an overview of MI and its causes and current MI assessments and treatments. Lastly, the use of art therapy for treating MI is discussed and several examples of appropriate directives are given.

MORAL INJURY
What is moral injury?

Litz *et al.* (2009) stated that moral injury (MI) "involves an act of transgression that creates dissonance and conflict because it violates assumptions and beliefs about right and wrong and personal goodness" (p.698). Utilizing Litz's previous work, Drescher *et al.* (2011) came up with the following definition of MI: "Disruption in an indivdual's confidence and expectations about one's own or others' motivation or capacity to behave in a just and ethical manner" (p.9). The authors stated that MI could occur when one has witnessed a perceived immoral act or has failed to stop an immoral act such as the death of others, causing suffering or pain to others, and being inhuman, depraved, or cruel.

Drescher *et al.* (2011) tested this definition by asking mental health clinicians, chaplains, and researchers to critically evaluate the construct. The study participants agreed that MI did occur as a result of wartime experiences, and resulted in behavioral, social, psychological, and spiritual problems. Other findings were that the concept of MI is useful and needed and the diagnostic criteria for post-traumatic stress disorder (PTSD) does not fully encompass MI. Lastly, the results showed that changes to the definition should be made.

A different definition of MI was offered by Shay (2012): a betrayal of what is considered right, by someone with legitimate authority, in a high stakes situation.

Dursun and Watkins (2018) pointed out that since morals are influenced by culture, potentially morally injurious events (PMIEs) will impact individuals in different ways.

Sources of moral injury

MI and war have always existed in tandem, but certain characteritics of wars are more likely to result in MI (Dursun & Watkins, 2018). Litz *et al.* (2009) identified the following as potentially causing MI: "witnessing the aftermath of violence and human carnage" (p.700) and "perpetrating, failing to prevent, bearing witness to, or learning about acts that transgress deeply held moral beliefs and expectations" (p.700). In 2013, Vargas *et al.* examined MI themes in the responses of Vietnam veterans to the National Vietnam Veterans' Readjustment Study. Results showed the following to be possible MI events: civilian death, within-ranks violence, other disproportionate violence, and betrayals.

Singer (2004) stated: "In the field, a solider must live up to the expectations of men he fights alongside of, even if that means committing atrocities, or he will feel ashamed" (p.381). However, while a soldier's actions may be justified by his military culture, he may still feel considerable distress due to how the actions go against his civilian morals (Schorr *et al.*, 2018). In 2016, Purcell *et al.* interviewed 26 combat veterans about the psychosocial impact of killing in war and found that for many veterans, killing was morally injurious. Wisco *et al.* (2017) found "a total of 10.8% of combat veterans acknowledged transgressions by self, 25.5% endorsed transgressions by others, and 25.5% endorsed betrayal" (p.340).

In 2018, Schorr *et al.* finally investigated the types of events that veterans viewed as morally injurious. The results were divided into two categories: personal responsibility and responsibility of others. Under personal responsibility, the following were considered sources of MI: harming civilians and civilian life, failing to prevent harm to others, killing or injuring the enemy in battle, and engaging in disproportionate violence. The responsibility of others category included: harming civilians and civilian life, witnessing or learning about immoral of unethical acts by trusted others, betrayal by systems (i.e. the military or the government), and witnessing or learning about disproportionate violence. Betrayal by trusted others and betrayal by systems were the categories most frequently mentioned by veterans (Schorr *et al.*, 2018).

IMPACT OF MORAL INJURY

Many researchers have investigated the impact of MI. Stein *et al.* (2012) found that MI was a predictor of guilt and re-experiencing symptoms. Yan (2016) found that MI not only impacts mental health, but it also negatively impacts physical health. Purcell *et al.* (2016) found that killing in war can impact individuals in many ways: questioning if justice or divinity exists when violence can take the lives of some but not others, questioning if they can be a good person again after killing, fear that the violence experienced during war may re-emerge, and difficulty integrating wartime experiences with post-war identity and worldview.

Wisco *et al.* (2017) examined MI in combat veterans using data from the National Health and Resilience in Veterans Study. Types of PMIEs were assessed using the Moral Injury Events Scale, and other established assessments were utilized to examine psychiatric and functional outcomes. Results indicated that transgressions by self are less common that other types of PMIEs but may be more damaging. Betrayal was found to be "significantly associated with postemployment suicide attempts" (Wisco *et al.*, 2017, p.345). PMIEs were also "associated with increased odds of current mental disorders and current suicidal ideation" (Wisco *et al.*, 2017, p.345).

MI ASSESSMENT

MI is a relatively new concept so there are not a lot of assessment options for clinicians. This also makes MI hard to study. Koenig, Youssef, and Pearce (2019) conducted a review of MI assessment instruments discussed in literature between 1980 and 2018. They found a total of five multi-dimensional scales: three which assess symptoms of MI and two which assess both MI events and symptoms.

Moral Injury Events Scale (MIES)

Nash *et al.* developed the Moral Injury Events Scale (MIES) in 2013. After a literature review, "a team of experts generated a pool of items generically describing events involving perpetrating, failing to prevent, bearing witness to, learning about, or being victim to acts that contradict deeply held beliefs and expectations" (Nash *et al.*, 2013, p.647). Consensus, testing on two cohorts of the Marine Resiliency Study, and tests for internal reliability and psychometric properties, resulted in nine items. Factor analysis of the nine items resulted in a two-factor solution: perceived transgressions by self or others and perceived betrayals by others. The data suggested that the MIES had good temporary stability (one week to three months), and supported construct validity.

Bryan *et al.* (2015) tested the psychometric properties of the MIES with a clinical sample of Air Force personnel and a non-clinical sample of Army National Guard personnel. The results of this study did not support the previous two-factor solution identified by Nash *et al.* (2013). Instead, results supported a three-factor solution: transgressions committed by self, transgressions committed by others, and perceived betrayals by others (Bryan *et al.*, 2015). The authors suggested adding additional items to the MIES, determining that MIES scores are responsive to clinical intervention, and investigating if the MIES is able to predict future emergence of depression, suicide risk, and PTSD. After reviewing MI assessments in 2019, Koenig *et al.* found that the MIES was "the most frequently used multidimensional measure in the literature that assess PMIEs and MI Symptoms" (p.9).

Moral Injury Questionnaire—Military Version (MIQ-M)

The year 2013 brought about another MI assessment, the Moral Injury Questionnaire—Military Version (MIS-M), developed by Currier *et al.* (2015). The MIQ-M is a 19-item self-reporting measure that assesses both causes and effects of potentially morally injurious events. The initial study by Currier *et al.* (2015) provided preliminary evidence for the validity of the MIQ-M.

In 2018, Braitman *et al.* conducted a test using a modified version of the MIQ-M in order to assess both morally injurious events (MIEs) and characteristics of MI such as guilt, shame, difficulties forgiving self and others, and withdrawal. Exploratory factor analysis for the modified MIQ-M found three factors: atrocities of war, psychological consequences of war, and leadership failure or betrayal. Results found that "exposure to MIEs and the defining characteristics MI…were moderately correlated with symptoms of anxiety, depression, and PTSD, such that more MIE exposure and associated characteristics were associated with worse mental health symptoms" (Braitman *et al.*, 2018, p.309). In 2019, Koenig *et al.* reported that the MIQ-M was the second most frequently used multidimensional scale in MI literature.

Moral Injury Symptoms Scale— Military Version (MISS-M)

One of the scales that measures MI symptoms, the MISS-M was developed by Koenig *et al.* (2018a) to address religious struggles or war-related changes in faith and in order to allow for tracking improvement in MI symptoms over time. The MISS-M consists of 45 items that make up ten subscales: shame, moral concerns, betrayal, guilt, loss of religious faith/hope, loss of meaning/purpose, religious struggles, difficulty for-giving, loss of trust, and self-condemnation. Results of initial studies show the MISS-M was reliable and valid and could be utilized to assess treatment outcomes for veterans and active duty military and to identify individuals who may be at risk of MI (Koenig *et al.*, 2018a). After developing the MISS-M, Koenig *et al.* (2018b) developed The Moral Injury Symptoms Scale—Military Version—Short Form (MISS-M-SF) that consists of ten questions, one for each of the subscales identified above. The authors reported, "The Miss-M-SF is internally reliable, temporally stable, and has acceptable construct validity, discriminate validity, and strong convergent validity with the original 45-item MISS-M" (Koenig *et al.*, 2018b, p.e663). The authors stated that the MISS-M-SF allows clinicians to quickly assess MI symptoms and can be used to monitor response to treatment.

Expressions of Moral Injury Scale— Military Version (EMIS-M)

Currier *et al.* (2017a) developed the EMIS-M to assess "the warning signs of MI in military populations" (p.474). The authors conducted two studies and found that the "EMIS-M is best conceptualized as two distinct but related factors" (p.484): expressions of MI directed at the self, and expression of MI directed at others. Study results also showed strong convergent and divergent validity. The EMIS-M can be used by clinicians to help determine appropriate course of treatment based on the individual's expression of MI (at self or others) (Currier *et al.*, 2017a).

TREATING MORAL INJURY

In developing a clinical care model for treatment of MI, Litz *et al.* (2009) worked under the assumption that MI is only possible when an individual has an intact moral belief system; "anguish, guilt, and shame are signs of an intact conscious and self- and other-expectations about goodness, humanity and justice" (p.701). Another assumption was that there were two routes that would allow for repair of a moral injury: "(a) psychological- and emotional-processing of the memory of the moral transgression, its meaning and significance, and the implication for the service member, and (b) exposure to corrective life experience" (Litz et al., p.701).

The treatment approach for MI developed by Litz et al. (2009) begins with establishing strong therapeutic rapport. Psychoeducation on MI and its impact are then provided. The third step in the process is an emotion-focused disclosure of the events that led to MI. Next, maladaptive beliefs about the self and the world are examined. Step number five involves having the client complete an empty chair dialogue with a benevolent moral authority. Making amends, or using good deeds as a vehicle to self-forgiveness, is step number six. During step seven, clients seek positive relationships outside therapy and are guided on how others may act if they share the cause of their MI. The final step is to look to the future and help clients establish realistic expectations about their recovery. The authors stated they realized that some steps would overlap and that some would likely occur throughout treatment.

Singer (2004) wrote about working with Vietnam veterans who had committed atrocities, and made five treatment recommendations. First, expressions of self-hatred should be allowed and eventually seen as an understandable emotion. Next, it is important to understand that many veterans will need to express remorse, self-hatred, and guilt throughout their life. The third recommendation is for therapists to avoid pushing forgiveness. Forgiveness comes from within and many develop this via atonement-like activities. Encouraging clients to re-connect with others is the fourth recommendation. Lastly, clients should be assisted in integrating before, during, and after war identities.

Adaptive disclosure (AD)

AD is a manualized treatment for PSTD as the result of traumatic loss, MI, or life-threatening/fear-based experiences (Steenkamp et al., 2011). AD was designed specifically for active service members. The treatment consists of six 90-minute individual sessions over the course of six weeks. The first session consists of psychoeducation. The next four sessions are exposure based; this allows for disproving negative expectations that many clients have about disclosing their traumatic experiences. The final session allows for future-oriented planning. The authors acknowledge that such a brief intervention is not likely to result in full symptom remission, but state that it is intended to teach patients coping skills and set them on a path towards healing. The briefness of the treatment is beneficial in that it allows busy service members to complete treatment quickly and, in the authors' view, would be more acceptable than non-time limited treatments. Additionally, military culture was considered and the authors stated that "AD is conceptualized as 'training' that will enhance the service member's effectiveness and performance by teaching him or her better ways of coping with and managing combat stress reactions" (Steenkamp *et al.*, 2011, p.101).

Adaptive disclosure is different from other treatments in that "the primary focus is promoting self-forgiveness and moving forward rather than disputing the rationality of appraisals about the nature of the act" (Gray *et al.*, 2012, p.410). AD also differs from other forms of treatment because it allows for treatment to focus on loss-based or MI-based PTSD. AD has been found to result in significant improvement in PTSD and depression symptoms, and significant decreases in negative beliefs about self and the world (Gray *et al.*, 2012).

Cognitive processing therapy (CPT) and prolonged exposure (PE)

Many authors suggest that current PTSD treatments may not be applicable to treating MI, however, Held *et al.* (2017) have found that CPT and PE can be effective treatments for those with MI-based PTSD. The authors published two case studies: one that utilized CPT and one that utilized PE to treat MI-based PTSD. In both cases, significant reduction in PTSD and depression symptoms was achieved. The authors believed that the improvements "were the result of confronting avoidance and adding greater levels of contextual detail to the traumatic memory, which helped these patients reappraise and restructure their original, erroneous interpretations of the events" (Held *et al.*, 2017, p.11). Although CPT and PE did help alleviate symptoms in the two cases reported, the authors acknowledge that treating MI-based PTSD can be more difficult and complex than treating other types of trauma.

Warrior Camp (WC)

Trauma and Resiliency Resources, Inc.'s WC is an intensive seven-day treatment which utilizes traditional and non-traditional treatment modalities, including yoga, equine-assisted psychotherapy (EAP), narrative writing, and eye movement desensitization and reprocessing therapy (Steele *et al.*, 2018). The authors assessed PTSD symptoms, depressive symptoms, relational attachment and MI. Results showed statistically significant differences (improvements) in pre- and post-treatment scores on all measurers. The authors suggested that EAP might help address the symptoms measured because "horses are able to give feedback about participants experience in a way that encourages thoughtful exploration and resolution" (Steele *et al.*, 2018).

Impact of killing (IOK)

IOK is a six- to eight-session treatment for MI that focuses on the act of killing and the distress experienced after combat (Purcell *et al.*, 2018a). IOK aims at self-forgiveness and asks veterans to consider how to create a life beyond suffering a shame while honoring their moral convictions. During treatment, barriers to treatment are discussed, "including the stigma and shame associated with talking about killing" (Purcell *et al.*, 2018a, p.651.) Discussions of killing are de-stigmatized via examination of common emotional, physiological, and cognitive responses to killing in combat. Between the second and third sessions, participants write a meaning statement about how killing has changed their beliefs about themselves, others, and the world. Later in treatment, the veteran defines self-forgiveness, identifies potential barriers to self-forgiveness, and works with the therapist to develop a "forgiveness plan." Next, veterans develop an amends plan that focuses on specific actions they can take. Treatment concludes with a chance to reflect on progress made during treatment and to make plans for continued work after treatment (Purcell *et al.*, 2018a).

Acceptance and commitment therapy (ACT)

ACT focuses on increasing social and behavioral functioning via identification and pursuit of personal values (Farnsworth *et al.*, 2017). The authors stated that when ACT is used to treat MI, veterans are encouraged to "view the emotional fallout of MI as informative rather than negative" (p.394); they studied the acceptability and feasibility of using ACT as a treatment for MI. Participants attended six 75-minute group sessions over two weeks and took part in post-group interviews. ACT was well tolerated by the participants and most had positive reactions to the treatment. Although the study sample was small, results were positive and indicate that further research should be conducted to determine if ACT is a truly effective treatment for MI (Farnsworth *et al.*, 2017).

BEST PRACTICES WHEN TREATING MI

Treating veterans and military service members with MI is similar in many ways to treating people from other cultures. Clinicians need to be culturally competent. Yan (2016) recommended that clinicians also become competent in addressing existential crises. Held *et al.* (2017) stressed the importance of non-judgment and acceptance from clinicians in order to avoid intensifying the MI or reinforcing the veteran's existing maladaptive beliefs.

Many researchers have commented on the desire of therapists to alleviate suffering, and how this desire may be counterproductive to helping someone with MI (Held *et al.*, 2017; Purcell *et al.*, 2016; Sullivan & Starnino, 2018). Purcell *et al.* (2016) stated that "some veterans want and need to sit with the incongruity between their actions in war and their own sense of morality and justice… Too readily minimizing the 'dark side'…may only deepen the disconnect between the veteran and clinician" (p.1091). Forgiveness is not always needed and is sometimes impossible or very difficult to obtain; forgiveness is "a deeply personal matter and one that often requires painful exploration of the consequences of one's actions and the harm done to others" (Purcell *et al.*, 2018).

Applying the principles of trauma-informed care (TIC) can help therapists ensure they are providing the best possible treatment for their clients (Currier *et al.*, 2017b). The first principle is safety and includes anything that impacts the physical environment of treatment as well as things that impact perceived emotional safety. The second principle is trustworthiness and includes clear communication and transparency from both the individual provider and the organization. Choice and collaboration are the third and fourth principles of TIC; therapists must consider the personal and cultural preferences of the client and allow them to be a partner in the treatment planning process. This "also compels providers to modify delivery of evidence-based interventions to adhere to veterans' needs and resources" (Currier *et al.*, 2017b, p.55). Lastly, therapists should help empower veterans by encouraging self-advocacy.

Art therapy

In the many MI articles I have read, only two addressed utilizing creative methods in treatment. Purcell *et al.* (2016) discussed the use of literature, theater, and humanities in treatment. "Unlike traditional therapy groups or PTSD groups, art and literature groups are not organized around a shared diagnosis or symptoms, but rather around a shared desire for creative exploration of the meaning of war's violence" (Purcell *et al.*, 2016, p.1092). The benefit of such groups is having a community of others who have had similar experiences, and having the opportunity to express thoughts and feelings in a new way. Art therapists can utilize these ideas when running programs for military veterans; groups can be focused around the idea of discussing war's impact on all facets of life. Participants can be encouraged to discuss the "hard stuff" while in a safe environment with a support system.

Creative methods for the treatment of MI were also championed by Schaff (2018). The author stated that telling others about one's experiences via narrative means such as poetry or stories is healing. This process requires the individual to take responsibility for "wrongs" done in the past, and "such writings offer the potential for healing those who suffer the moral wounds of war" (Schaff, 2018, p.132). If telling one's story is beneficial, then it is likely that reading poems or stories written by others could contribute to healing.

Art therapy directives

Although there are no articles that specifically address using art therapy to treat MI, creative activities are present in many articles that address MI treatment or PTSD treatments and mention MI. In discussing ACT as a treatment for MI, Farnsworth *et al.* (2017) detailed a values-based activity in which clients write a word symbolizing their most distressing MIE on one side of a rock, and a word that symbolizes a personal value that was violated during the MIE but that they wish to uphold moving forward in life, on the other side of the rock. The authors stated that the rock symbolizes the connection between values and suffering in MI and that "allowing" the memory and pain associated with violation of a value are necessary in order to continue to have this value (Farnsworth *et al.*, 2017). This exercise could be utilized as described, or clients could create images that represent the MIE and the value violated.

Lobban and Murphy (2019) detailed the use of art therapy in treating veterans with chronic PTSD. Two of the directives mentioned in the article may be useful when treating MI, with minor adjustment. First, veterans could create two images: 1) the MIE; and 2) current emotional responses when under stress. This exercise may help veterans be less judgmental of the choices they made at the time of the MIE, while at the same time enabling an understanding of how perceptions have been impacted. Second, veterans could create images to depict the lived experience of MI.

Another directive that could be used to treat MI was provided to me by Debra Rogers (personal communication, August 24, 2020). She has utilized masks in group treatment of veterans with MI. Prompts include considering what could be taken away and what could be added to one's life; showing one's values and beliefs, and how one understands the world; focusing on a poignant experience and how that changed their views of themselves, others, the world, and their spirituality. Once the veteran has created the mask, discussions can focus on how their values have changed as a result of their experiences or how their mask might change as a result of what they have heard and seen throughout the group mask-making process.

Jones has used celebration/commemoration boxes when working with veterans with traumatic brain injury and psychological health conditions like PTSD (Mims & Jones, 2019); "Service members are invited to create a box or container in which the outside of the box celebrates aspect of career and self and the inside of the box commemorates or memorizes aspects of career, self, and/or buddies lost" (p.324). This directive could be used in the treatment of MI as well by focusing on changes to one's values and identity as a result of the traumatic experiences. Many who are dealing with MI also have survivors' guilt and it would be appropriate to utilize the box to address this as well.

CONCLUSION

Although there is not currently very much literature on the treatment of MI, especially from a creative or art therapy standpoint, more and more articles are published each year. Several directives that are currently being used in the field have been highlighted. Like those mentioned, other directives could easily be changed to be appropriate for use with those suffering from MI. Once we become familiar with MI and its impact on veterans and military service members, we can adapt our current practices to meet the needs of these individuals.

Chapter 7

Mission Resiliency: A Large-Group Art Therapy Program

— DEBORAH MURPHY —

INTRODUCTION TO MISSION RESILIENCY

A group art therapist performs a valuable service and holds a unique position in an institution. When art therapy is navigated with a clear mission, the rewards are innumerable. For the most part, whether the setting is school-based, medical or psychiatric, non-profit, private or governmental, a central element to all is the bringing together of individuals for the purpose of art making for therapy. This chapter describes how I developed an inpatient active-duty art therapy program in a private psychiatric hospital. I share how my theoretical applications, experience, and passion for this profession have contributed to a solid program. This chapter is about my particular experience working with service members who have come to treatment for reoccurring suicidal thoughts or attempts. Trauma symptoms or substance abuse may have taken such a toll on their relationships that treatment may be a last resort or ultimatum to save a marriage and family. They may find themselves admitted as an order from their command or from failure to improve in an outpatient setting. The reasons are numerous. I am an art therapist who relies on the power of group process to reach over 650 active-duty service members in all branches of our armed forces annually. I am an art therapist who knows that, if willing, any one service member can find a way to make meaning from their participation in art therapy groups. Their results may be life altering or simply provide acknowledgement that there is a way to engage pleasurably with others through mutual arts participation. I would like to give recognition and honor to all by sharing what I have come to find helpful through this chapter.

Mission Resiliency is the active-duty treatment program for which I manage art therapy services, alongside other patient population programs at Laurel Ridge Treatment Center (LRTC) in San Antonio, Texas. It celebrated its tenth year in 2019, and I was tasked to ask Mission Resiliency patients to submit art for an annual calendar because it was clear that the artistic expressions created by our service members were powerful. With the proper releases in place, a calendar was printed for distribution to the public, patients, and their families.

Before I explain more about the program, I want to acknowledge all the staff and department heads who have been a tremendous support to my work on so many levels. I thank my immediate co-workers who help keep my groups safe, encourage our service members to attend art therapy groups, follow up patient art projects to completion, or simply validate their work in the making. I want to shout out to the nurse manager who has been the ultimate coach and kept my vision clear. Our clinical manager is creative and passionate about our program. She has a vision and understands how art can contribute to healing our patients. All these individuals have been advocates for art therapy and instrumental in ensuring that our new building, which opened in October 2020, included a large art studio space and that each patient wing was given an area in which to make art.

When the active-duty program was in the planning stages at my workplace, I had been a full-time group art therapist for the child, adolescent, and adult psychiatric inpatient units. I saw veterans on occasion in my regular adult substance abuse and mood disorder programs. Their art and stories were remarkable, and I saw purpose in the group service I provided. I felt I needed to be in this new program named "Mission Resiliency." There have been many therapists before me who have treated military personal with art therapy and described the impact and positive change within this community. I was just another witness to this phenomenon. I brought art from the veterans in my groups with their stories to the program developers. They were easily convinced that my specific skill set would be beneficial and I was welcomed. My first challenge was finding a physical space to have a studio-based program in a building that was not designed for that purpose. This problem is not unique to most art therapists. I made it work by virtue of persistence, creativity, and humor.

Originally, the Laurel Ridge Mission Resiliency program was a 60-bed treatment program situated on a campus alongside child, adolescent, and adult psychiatric programs totaling 250 beds. It is one of the largest behavioral health hospitals in Texas and the nation. Mission Resiliency is dynamic and continues to seek new methods to improve. Because of its successful evidence-based outcomes, this program expanded to 80 beds in a state-of-the-art facility across the street from the 18-acre Laurel Ridge campus.

> The Mission Resiliency program is structured using Substance Abuse and Mental Health Services Administration, evidence-based curriculums, clinical outcome data, Department of Defense (DoD) medication/diagnosis protocol and the Total Force Fitness Model. The fidelity of this program is continually audited internally and externally to ensure the effectiveness of the resiliency mission. (Laurel Ridge Treatment Center, 2020)

Primary treatments include cognitive behavioral therapy, prolonged exposure, and cognitive processing therapy. These services are established in all programs that include combat trauma, military sexual trauma, substance abuse, and dual diagnosis. Therapists are certified in prolonged exposure therapy and are given supervision with national experts. Other treatment modalities include:

- Reintegration outings
- Daily physical training, sports courts, resistance machines, and free weights

- Weekly patient leadership meetings
- Spiritual services (optional)
- Primary care medical doctors are available
- Psychiatrist daily visits
- Specialized Therapeutic Services: Art Therapy, Therapeutic Recreation, Music Therapy, and a ROPES course (Repetitive Obstacle Performance Evaluation System)
- Yoga
- Massages
- Animal-assisted therapy
- Aquatic therapy
- Virtual reality technology (when indicated)
- Denial management
- Education on disease process
- Relapse prevention
- Shame and survivors' guilt support
- Alcoholics Anonymous
- Narcotics Anonymous
- Education groups (i.e. mindfulness, confidence building, stress reduction, seeking safety)
- Military-specific groups (topics relate to life stressors and issues unique to military personnel).

Prolonged exposure therapy (PE), a key component to combat trauma and non-combat trauma tracks, teaches individuals to gradually approach their trauma-related memories, feelings, and events through imaginal and in-vivo experiences that expose patients to things and places they normally would avoid because of trauma symptoms (Levine, 1997; Najavits, 2002). Art therapy has enabled service members to use visual arts media to explore their trauma as an extension of PE. It has also given individuals the opportunity to release tension or explore the multitude of other therapeutic benefits that will be detailed in later in this chapter.

ART THERAPY TRAINING AND BACKGROUND EXPERIENCE

The nature versus nurture debate resonates clearly in the development of any art therapist with nearly 40 years of practice. Our academic training gives us the soil and nutrients to feed our roots. Life and employment influence us throughout the rest of our career. Our basic resilience lets us see where we survive and where we thrive. Some of us write about it, teach about it, support policies about it, or continue to apply it to the individuals and groups we serve. Some of us do bit of all these things.

I have always felt the artist in me. My family nurtured this more than in any other practical direction. As a result, I pursued a liberal arts education with a degree in fine arts and a minor in secondary art education. I went directly into the art therapy program at Wright State University, Dayton, Ohio. Department Head, Dr. Gary Barlow, then Editor of the *American Art Therapy Journal*, with assisting instructors Dr. Louis Shupe and Virginia Niswander, opened my eyes to the world of art therapy in the early 1980s. They invited renowned national art therapists, such as Harriet Wadeson, Janie Ryan, Robert Ault and Edward Adamson, to our classroom. We spent the summers learning about other expressive therapies with music, dance, and psychodrama. I gained practical experience with special needs military dependents in a program called CHAP (Children Have A Potential), spearheaded by Ms. Niswander on Wright Patterson Base.

I attained Ohio certification in special education with a plan to continue with this population. Instead, I had a seamless lift-off from internship in a state psychiatric institution to a full-time job where I had free rein and space to establish multiple art studios for painting, drawing, fiber arts, and ceramics. I added part-time work as a junior high school art teacher for a special education department, and that led me to a new full-time endeavor as an elementary school art teacher. My art therapy training was valuable in working with this underserved community in the inner city. Managing an art class in this climate was less than ideal and I had to quickly learn how to motivate positive behaviors to survive. Part-time work at the Dayton Art Institute at the same time kept me balanced and refreshed. Four years later, I was awarded a grant to do collaborative research with the art therapy department at Wright State University. Through a series of multimedia directives given to kindergarten students, we looked for specific indicators to identify academic at-risk factors. I left this research project to marry and start a family in San Antonio. Later, I re-entered clinical art therapy work. I found employment readily at inpatient, outpatient, and private child, adolescent, and adult psychiatric settings, community centers, geriatric psychiatric hospitals and day treatment programs, a charter school, cancer treatment centers, summer camps and finally at my current place of employment. I entered the counseling program at Our Lady of the Lake University to supplement my education and meet criteria to become a Licensed Professional Counselor in Texas. There were only a few other art therapists in the area and very little was known about it. I developed a passion for educating the public about art therapy.

I have been active in art therapy professional organizations since graduate school. From the Buckeye Art Therapy Association to the South Texas Art Therapy Association, I gained valuable mentorship, support, continuing education, and friendship that helped me broaden my scope of practice. It contributed to my identity as an art therapist in the company of other health professionals. My artist identity was always active. Out of graduate school, I acquired a kiln and potter's wheel. I made clay pots and sculptures, painted, and created art through fiber arts and mixed media. I have been commissioned to paint murals at four treatment centers and at a neighborhood community center.

At present, my mission is to expand art therapy in south Texas through my supervisory relationships with graduate, ATR, ATR-Provisional and Licensed Professional Counselor Interns working towards licensure with a specialty in art therapy. I continue my commitment to improving our profession through service on the Art Therapy Credentials Board. My nature to work hard, a strong sense of commitment and passion for art, and the nurture gained from art therapy colleagues were what led me to develop a strong military art therapy program and become the sole art therapist at one of the largest psychiatric hospitals in Texas.

ART THERAPY PROGRAM IDEOLOGY AND APPLICATION

When I was asked to write this chapter, I tried to look to the theory and art therapy approaches I apply most to this military population. I have always relied on developmental theory and the work from Eric Erikson's psychosocial stages. In identifying these stages, Erikson presents the struggles and issues one must overcome to successfully move on to the next. Themes of identity, intimacy, life, and work are common in my art therapy groups, with individuals ranging in age from their early 20s to late 40s. My respected colleague, Vicki Williams Patterson, explained my work from another perspective. When I take a closer look to compare my typical interactions with patients in an art therapy setting I can appreciate her suggestions that infer that I use phenomenological and art-based applications. I can make clear associations with Cathy Moon's (2002) studio art therapy descriptions in her book. Dr. Moon writes about relational aesthetics, "An art based model of art therapy highly values the artistic identity in both the therapist and the client" (Moon, 2002, pp.8–9) Generally, service members who come to my groups know that I am a therapist but they do not come with an intention to talk treatment issues with me or to be analyzed. Many only listen long enough to my opening art directive presentation to get a gist of what "they are supposed to do"; hence I provide a descriptive handout with a written feedback option. They call me an art teacher or expert. I am grateful for my fine arts education and having the bachelor's degree is respected in this community. I also feel fortunate to have relationships with professional artists who relate to me as an artist and advise me along the way. Those experiences have fueled the passion I try to impart to each patient. Even though there are cases where a patient comes to my group reluctantly and only out of compliance, I make it clear to them that engaging at some level with an art medium is worth trying.

I often follow similar sequences to those described in Betensky's (1987) phenomenological approach in a typical group by providing the space in which the patient can make art, directing the patient to distance themselves and look intentionally at their work; then finally, I ask the questions, "What do you see?" "What is the message?" (Betensky, 1987, pp.158–159). When I present a medium or topic for the session, I always give open-ended options to follow. This speaks to the patient-centered approach. The group makeup typically contains a few patients arriving for the first time and those ready for discharge, averaging 16–20 participants. This approach helps meet the varying needs of the milieu. Some patients appreciate my plans, handouts, demonstration, examples, and rationale. Some come to session with their own plan and simply tolerate my opening respectfully. Some, but few, come with a book to read. Some come in physical or emotional distress, too distracted to engage in any activity. For most, their genuine intent is to make something meaningful and aesthetically satisfying. What I try to impart is that the creative process and skill required to meet their high personal expectations may not be what they need. I give suggestions that promote exploration, self-acceptance, and understanding that art making needs to encompass all forms and levels, each having value. Squeezing clay or covering a canvas with color is just as worthy as making something to keep or give to another person. This is a difficult concept for most but an important building block in making the connections with mind, body, and spirit essential to healing from trauma or substance abuse recovery (Rubin, 1987).

The importance of presenting media variety to our service members has been one of my top priorities in art therapy groups. In line with Kagin and Lusebrink's (Hinz, 2009) expressive therapies continuum or Hass-Cohen and Findlay's (2013) art therapy relational neuroscience approach, the sensory, kinesthetic, controlled, and fluid properties of the art materials activate neurological systems crucial in healing trauma or managing symptoms of depression and anxiety. These researchers and others have written extensively on this topic and are able to articulate this process more clearly.

Speaking simply as a clinician, I believe that to know oneself better through art, a varied media exploration is an essential part of the art therapy process. When individuals experiment with different media and learn through trial and error, the whole brain is accessed, consequently unlocking the door to self-awareness. When the door is unlocked in a group setting, a ripple effect of internal and external interactions comes into play. The service members discover how art making can address their immediate internal needs—to reduce anxiety and trauma symptoms, to communicate difficult feelings and thoughts with a therapist, peers, or family members, to relieve stress, to explore interests, or to revisit positive memories, to name a few. Making art in the company of peers gives each service member feedback in the form of compliments, advice on their work, creative ways to elaborate, and humorous conversation. The group process also provides validation and empathy that trauma, depression, and addiction themes are understood and shared. Most often, the social aspect of making art in a community or among peers increases their bond or trust. Given that the composition of the groups changes weekly, with new admissions coming in and individuals discharging, it is common to hear reports from service members that it was the time in the art therapy group that gave them the opportunity to get to know each another better. This is well supported in Stephen Porges' (2019) polyvagal theory. Dr. Porges states: "Social behaviors are neural exercises that promote neurophysiological states supporting mental and physical health" (Porges, 2019, p.13).

WEEKLY ART THERAPY GROUPS—
THE MILITARY MILIEU

The treatment setting in which I work follows the medical model. We refer to all individuals receiving treatment as patients. I use the term "service members" and "patients" interchangeably in this chapter as a distinction. The Mission Resiliency units include three general tracks: combat trauma, non-combat trauma/military sexual trauma, and substance abuse disorders. Patients may have a mood disorder diagnosis and many are treated in dual programs. Patients with severe depression may receive electroconvulsive therapy. Combat trauma patients may have a traumatic brain injury.

My typical work week includes mandatory, two-hour art therapy groups and art workshops that are optional sessions for the active duty patients who have special projects or appreciate coming to the art room to create for relaxation or sharpen a skill. The dynamics of my work-load is always subject to change. Prior to the opening of the Mission Resiliency building, I served the entire civilian adult and active duty populations, that is, nine distinct programs. Currently, I treat the service members on four units at Mission Resiliency and the Military Partial Hospitalization Program, (PHP). I also hold groups twice weekly for the veterans' program on the Laurel Ridge Treatment Center main campus.

The years of experience working with individuals on the contin-uum of mental illnesses treated for severe psychosis, debilitating mood disorders, to life-threatening addictions undergoing detoxification protocols has been invaluable, particularly in recognizing the red flags with in-patient service members during art therapy sessions. For that reason, tools and sharps are always accounted for and images created that suggest at-risk behaviors are taken seriously and reported. On occasion, a service member may be transferred directly to the more restrictive civilian units because of an episode of psychosis, voicing suicidal thoughts or a display of self-harming behaviors.

The content of my art therapy groups vary dramatically from the days I worked with the civilian population to now as a sole provider for the military and veterans. As the civilians' typical length of stay is five to seven days, directives were structured wherein the whole group followed one theme. The media and tools were limited, with a higher emphasis on safety. I also facilitated an organized 30-minute formal verbal group process after each art-making experience. My goal was to educate on art therapy as an option for out-patient treatment in the community after discharge and as an alternative to voice difficult feelings and thoughts. I provided art therapy and art-based community resources and groups such as Open Art Studio and Visual Art Journaling.

In contrast, my military art therapy groups differ remarkably in theme and media from week to week. Janice Lobban (2017) refers to the military population as unique. She writes that "cultural characteristics moulded by military training, experiences surrounding exposure to military operations and combat, and breaking of secure attachments when leaving the military" are factors that need to be understood in effective treatment (Lobban, 2017, p.73). My rationale is to capture the attention of the masses quickly. Given that groups have an average of 16–20 participants, one must work quickly to keep all members engaged at some level and present the expectation that participation is an important element to the total treatment program. A typical service member may not view art therapy participation in the same way as the talk therapy and psychoeducation sessions, perhaps seeing it as optional. A common reason to decline art therapy is the perspective "I'm not artsy." I see this as a challenge and learning opportunity to educate each reluctant member about art therapy and its benefits. My tactics in confronting these individuals vary, based on intuition. I am mindful to check myself before approaching the non-compliant patient so my approach maintains empathy and professionalism. To encourage compliance, my clinical director suggested I teach a separate psych-education group on how art making effects brain function and its relationship with healing trauma. This has been an effective way for service members who struggle with coming to group to see my role as more than an "arts and crafts lady."

Art therapy groups have a consistent structure with flexibility. A group therapist must accept the less than ideal situations that happen daily. Some patients arrive late or are taken out of a session to see the psychiatrist or individual therapist. A service member from another unit may interrupt the group as a curious passerby or approach me with a personal request, not knowing a better time to reach me. I have learned some effective ways to manage this disruption. New members receive a written protocol to introduce them quickly to the session. This protocol includes a brief definition of art therapy, how to maintain safety and supplies, the general group timeline within the allotted two-hour period, what they may encounter creating art, and how to access help. I open each session with the theme and art directive. It is distributed with a handout that includes thematic quotes or a poem, the objective and possible outcome, a brief "how-to" sequence, and a process survey. This handout helps in a large group where members may feel at a loss as to where to begin. Clear direction is in line with military training. The confident, experienced, and self-directed participants serve as role models for the less secure. They may take on the role as the art therapy space tour guide or even do a little teaching.

The process survey on the handout has been the most practical method of assessing the service members' response to the intervention. Many group members would prefer to keep the art they make private. Others lack the language to verbalize what they have created. I have tried a variety of ways to keep the "process" in the group. Group members' engagement varies from being social and superficially involved to being totally focused, present, and in the flow. Stopping the art experience to facilitate a whole large-group verbal process has its challenges. When groups peak at larger numbers, the content of the discussion is easily sidetracked to be less than productive. Grandstanding, poking fun at one another, and minimizing the content of the art work can often take over and leave a disappointing end to an otherwise meaningful art experience. Characteristically, service members in this setting are not ready to speak genuinely about their experience in a large company of peers. This takes maturity and a universal sense of trust and acceptance. However, I have had some powerful disclosures over the years during one-on-one conversations within the group setting.

Before the opening of the stand-alone Mission Resiliency building, art therapy groups were held in an open day are to accommodate the average 16-25 patient attendees. The group art room designated for these sessions only fit 8-10 individuals. The advantage of this set up was patients could choose between a quite room or larger bustling area. However, it was not a closed safe space to share in a collective or to disclose thoughts and feelings privately. It was particularly disadvantageous to our population with combat trauma. Due to the successful response our services members had to the art therapy program voiced by therapists and managers, and as indicated on patient exit surveys, the administration implemented an art room with ample space and equipment with the expansion of the new building. Showcases were installed in the cafeteria and patient unit day areas to present patient artwork from those who want to share the impact this program had for them. It has been a way to communicate their story of hope and resilience gained by asking for help and coming to the realization they are not alone. Proper releases have been put into place to allow these products to be displayed. Additionally, our combat trauma program holds group therapy in what is called, "The War Room." The walls of this room have been covered with visual depictions of the wounds of wars, personal trauma events, inspirational and spiritual images, and pictures that give evidence of resolution. Written feedback enables participants to communicate on a more genuine level while allowing me to be available to those who need my help at the last minute. The written feedback is reviewed and, when appropriate, may prompt me to meet individually with a service member. I offer an option to return feedback forms for their own keeping. Many prefer to have their art and writings stored with me.

During the start of the session, once the handouts are distributed, I present the topic with historical and cultural references, visual examples, and a demonstration. I find putting the art directive in universal terms provides an acceptable rationale to make art for self. For example, cave paintings were designed to communicate stories, resilience is found in nature, cultural traditions honor the deceased, a mandala is used for prayer, ritual, and meditation. In most cases, I offer a choice of materials to carry out the themes and directives. Again, bearing in mind that this work is done with a large group, this approach keeps the invitation to make art open and available. Many service members have an idea of what they want to do before coming. A rigid approach can quickly turn a session into a power struggle.

Some patients need the sensory comfort of modeling clay, while others want the control to draw with a graphite pencil. The general expectation is to try different media at some point over the course of the four to six weeks of treatment. This mirrors how talk therapists encourage patients to change behaviors. Working through the awkwardness or discomfort of a particular art medium is a safe way to practice new behaviors, facilitating growth and new perspectives. When I suggest new media approaches, I make it clear to each individual that this is only a suggestion. They must trust their instincts and strive to recognize what outcomes are needed to succeed in treatment. In most cases, the service member knows what is needed to progress. The challenge is to do the work. My role is to identify what will help them move forward, using one-to-one consultation during the sessions through the weeks (Csamanski-Cohen & Weihs, 2016; Wilkinson & Chilton, 2013).

My group directives are dynamic. They evolve to meet current group needs and my exposure to new trends, art techniques, and cultural learning. This personally challenges and energizes my professional work, and keeps patients with extended stays or those who have had to return to treatment curious about what they may do next. Unlike the set curriculum in psychoeducation groups, I have the freedom to create my interventions. Patients often ask me, "What do you have planned for art therapy?" Healing needs inquisitiveness as an important element for growth. Still, over the many years this program has been in existence, I have certain interventions and media applications that are particularly effective from a whole-group perspective. I change the media week to week from fluid to controlled, sensory to less provocative. Like an effective physical workout, moving from two dimensional to three dimensional, soft to aggressive applications, colorful to neutral, these interventions work the whole brain. Through written processes, the service members are asked what they were mindful of during art making and how one medium differed from another. They are asked which materials are comforting and which ones may be frustrating. These conversations lead to self-insights and areas to explore.

SAMPLE DIRECTIVES
VISUAL IMAGERY USING DOORS

Objective: Patient will identify challenges, opportunities past, present, and future that impact treatment goals.

Motivational quote: "When one door closes, another opens: but we often look so long and so regretfully upon the closed door that we do not see the one which has opened for us." (Alexander Graham Bell)

Task: Draw or paint a series of doors that represent different challenges and opportunities. Create a setting for these doors that is either inside or outside. Visualize each door with as much detail as possible. What color, size, and shape are these doors? Are there decorations or signs, are they accessible or difficult to enter? Elaborate on this in your setting/ environment that you imagine (Capacchione, 1989, p.16).

Options: Sculpt this scene or create a sign for a door that represents something you would like to welcome in your life. Draw or construct a self-portrait in the likeness of Janus the Roman God of doors to reflect what you want to let go from the last year and an intention for the in-coming year (this directive may be introduced in January to coincide with new year's resolutions).

Supplies: Drawing-pencils, rulers and stencils, 12" x 18" quality paper, carbon paper to transfer images from therapist's collection (includes different doors, e.g., revolving, Dutch, sliding, glass, elevator, saloon, medieval), acrylics, brushes, canvas boards, clay, rolling pins and clay tools.

Process survey questions:

1. What challenges and opportunities did you represent?
2. Did you notice any thoughts or feelings while depicting any of these doors?
3. Other comments?

MASK WE WEAR

Objective: Given examples and brief history of mask-making and their functions, patient to understand the therapeutic benefit of catharsis through active mask-making.

Motivational quote: "Man is least himself when he talks in his own person. Give him a mask, and he will tell you the truth." (Oscar Wilde)

Task: Use the plastic mold, model clay and/or adhere other three-dimensional forms to produce a character. It may have human, animal, alien, mythical, or any other elements. Apply plaster gauze over your forms, paint when plaster has set, and add mixed media if desired (fur, feathers, shells, and other found objects). If desired, mount on a canvas board to create a setting for this mask.

Options: Masks versus true identity. Contrast the mask with how you present yourself to others on the outside, with your true self on the inside of the mask. Magazine images may be included.

Supplies: Plastic forms, clay, cardboard, and masking tape to adhere form for hand building, plaster gauze (preferred medical supply stores over art supply companies). For finishing: acrylic paints, brushes, canvas boards, and mixed media.

Process survey questions:

1. What feelings, thoughts, and visceral responses were you mindful of when constructing the mask?
2. What would you name your mask or what emotion/character does it portray to you?
3. If your mask were to speak this sentence, how would it be completed? "I am the one who..."
4. Other comments?

▧ WATERCOLOR

Objective: Patient practices the principle of "letting go" with spontaneous watercolor exploration.

Motivational quote: "Empty your mind, be formless, shapeless—like water. Now you put water in a cup, it becomes the cup; put water in a bottle, it becomes the bottle; you put water in a teapot, it becomes the teapot. Now water can flow or it can crash. Be water my friend." Bruce Lee

Task: Tape watercolor paper into four sections; follow the demonstration using watercolors with saran wrap, oil pastels, sponge application, and salt.

Follow-up options: Remove the tape and in the open spaces write words of inspiration. Using the techniques learned, create another painting that expresses: my emotions, like a body of water; a road that illustrates my journey and where I want to go; the four elements (fire, water, earth and air).

Supplies: Watercolor paper and board to tape it down, watercolors, brushes, sponges, masking tape of varying thickness, oil pastels, and salt.

Process survey questions:

1. What were your successes and/or struggles with this medium? Any discoveries?
2. What theme did you use? How does it relate to your treatment?
3. Other comments?

WHAT I HOLD DEAR

Objective: Patient will draw, paint or sculpt hands in an art form that identifies what they hold dear, and is one motivation for treatment.

Motivational reference: "When things get out of control, we say they are out of hand. When we want to take control, we try to get a grip, or get a handle on things. When we are missing a view of fundamental reality, we say we are out of touch. When we are likely to say something truthful, but possibly embarrassing, our mothers tell us to sit on our hands. Hands can reveal vocations. Gestures communicate thoughts and feelings. Hands reveal emotions, for example tapping, sweaty palms." (Retrieved from http://wisdomofhands.blogspot.com/2009/09/hands-as-metaphor-for-control.html)

Task: Trace your hands in a drawing, painting, or slab of clay. Create an image that represents something you hold dear or what it is you are reaching for.

Supplies: Drawing-pencils, rulers and stencils, 12" x 18" quality paper, carbon paper to transfer images from internet images, acrylics, brushes, canvas boards, clay, rolling pins, and clay tools.

Process survey questions:

1. What does your art represent?
2. What did you find beneficial or not so beneficial?
3. Other comments?

CONTAINERS

Objective: Patient to construct a container to instill hope or symbolize another need.

Motivational quote: "A cup of tea is a cup of peace." Unknown source.

Task: Having received the handout with examples of various containers, construct a container that represents something you need, such as hope, inspiration, love, focus, nurturance, peace. The demonstration includes slab hand building construction and methods to apply to a coffee cup (focus), a candle holder (peace or to memorialize someone), a goblet (spiritual search), a soup bowl or pot for a plant (nurturance).

Options: Bottled feelings or your black box (i.e., construct a box that represents you). The output and input are seen, but the internal workings are not. Associations may include a computer, engine, or human brain.

Supplies: Clay, rolling pins, patterns for containers, clay tools, stamps and cookie cutters to create surface designs.

Process survey questions:

1. What kind of container did you make and why?
2. What thoughts or feelings were you mindful of when constructing in clay?
3. Other comments?

CHAOS EXAMINED

Objective: Learn how a creative process can access internal messages.

Motivational reference: Today's theme is "Creating Chaos". Normally, we tend to flee from disorder and chaos; identifying chaos with evil and destruction. It may be suggested that looking at chaos may be a way of gaining wisdom. (Marshall, 2011).

Task: Choose items from the table of recycled and found objects that catch your attention, without making judgments. Arrange and attach items to the canvas board in a manner that represents your chaos. Keep in mind appropriate glues for different materials.

Supplies: Wide variety of found and recycled objects, recycled canvas boards, white glue, Mod Podge®, hot glue, scissors, and tape.

Process survey questions:

1. How did you choose the collage materials?
2. Distancing yourself from your collage, describe your work with a title or phrase.
3. What wisdom can you gain from what you see?

HOW MEDIA INFLUENCES EMOTIONAL EXPRESSION

Objective: Patient to experience and compare how three contrasting mediums effect how expressing a feeling in art as a method to practice mindfulness.

Motivational reference: Today's objective is to practice mindfulness while using different art materials. Mindfulness is an awareness of oneself in the present, recognizing thoughts, feelings and body sensations calmly without judgement. (Mindfulness is taught regularly in all program psych-education groups.) At the end, you will report how the different media affected you differently. You may be able to recognize what material may help with a particular symptom or issue you need to explore.

Task: Choose one feeling you want to explore. The feeling chosen may be one you struggle with or one you want to feel. Make three works of art that describe this feeling. 1. Draw the feeling in a word picture with pencils and graph paper. 2. Make a clay symbol of this feeling, such as an animal, thing, or abstraction. 3. Paint an abstraction of the feeling (no words or specific images).

Therapist's note: Due to the complexity of the task, visual examples are given for each medium. Abstract paintings and sculptures from Art History books give patients an idea of how color, energy of a brush stroke and shape project feeling states. This intervention pushes the patient to try new techniques they may not have been willing to use before.

Supplies: Clay, clay tools, acrylic paints, brushes, 5" x 7" canvas boards, graphite pencils, rulers, stencils, erasers, and graph paper.

Process survey questions:

1. How is the feeling you chose relevant to you right now?
2. Did you experience different reactions to using different media?
3. Viewing your three artworks, which medium best describes the feeling you chose. Which medium were you most comfortable with?

MANDALAS AND MINDFULNESS

Objective: Practice mindfulness through mandala drawing using dominant and sub-dominant hands.

Motivational quote: Each person's life is like a mandala—a vast, limitless circle. We stand in the center of our own circle, and everything we see, hear and think forms the mandala of our life." (Saraha)

Task: Using oil pastels or chalk pastel, fill the circle on white paper with colors and shapes, using your dominant hand. Follow the same instruction with a second drawing on black paper, using your sub-dominant hand.

Process survey questions:

1. Look at your picture from all four angles, choose the best view, and write the date at the bottom of the picture.
2. Look at the parts. What part do you like and what part not so much? How about the whole? Does it remind you of something or do you have a felt sense about it?
3. Write down these observations. Give your drawings a title. Note thoughts, feelings, and body responses you experienced when drawing with each hand (Fincher, 1989; Kellogg, 1984).

CLAY AND KILN FIRING

The introduction of clay hand building to service members has been an indispensable component of the group art therapy experience. Many non-artists find drawing a negative experience difficult and default immediately to their lack of skill, a perception that obstructs the ability to focus on the content and meaning of their expression. This is especially true in the company of peers, as military personnel commonly are competitive and dislike exposing their weaknesses. Clay, however, is malleable and forgiving. The pulling, squeezing, and rolling kinesthetic movements provide an immediate release of tension, anxiety, and aggression, distracting one from such insecurities. Depressed patients find solace in sculpting and creating a product. The scope of work I've encountered is truly remarkable. From a simple ashtray to a complex sculpture depicting a post-traumatic stress disorder (PTSD) brain or a Spartan helmet, the vast majority of patients have found something that resonates within them in this medium. Clay brings people together and at the same time gives an individual a space for solitude. As patients build self-reliance in understanding clay properties through manipulation and practice, they intuitively make products that meet their needs, both immediate and longer term (Anderson, 1995; Nan, 2016;Wong & Au, 2019).

For example, when Robert came to art therapy for the first time he looked depressed and anxious, hunched over, with poor eye contact. His dual diagnosis included PTSD and an addiction to opiates. He was given a lump of clay and guided demonstration on constructing two pinch pots to form an egg. Using the metaphor of the egg, he was asked to create something new. He fashioned a crude open box. The next week's topic was to draw, paint, or construct a box that represents what is hidden from others (i.e., black box theory). Robert wanted to use clay again and was shown how to build a slab box. He worked with more skill and confidence. He made a jewelry box for his wife and was pleased with his improvements. In the process survey he wrote: "This helped lower my anxiety. It reminded me how I have been numb and how it has affected me and the people around me." The short-term need was symptom management and to recognize his feelings of guilt and remorse. His long-term need was to show his wife that he treasures her even though he has not displayed these feelings. Many patients find making something for their loved one is a comfort during this separation. The product is a tangible way to connect and show how much they care.

Service members who get "hooked" on clay have the opportunity to work on their respective units. Large storage rooms were converted into unit art rooms stocked with art supplies available during free time. Some find the flow of building sculptures a way to manage the long hours in treatment, particularly in the evenings. Patients who encounter a difficult individual therapy session or spend time listening to their prolonged exposure tapes required in this mode of trauma treatment find that time in the art room gives them a breathing space to wind down. Creative talents are uncovered during this time alone from groups. It is like the opening of the unknown cell in Johari's Window. Sculptures often represent their faith, things their children and wives like, or what their PTSD looks like to them, in the likeness of demons, nightmares, trauma memories, or their brain. The image shown below (Figure 7.1) is an example of one service member's symbolic self-portrait. His skull is wrapped with the tentacles of a monstrous squid. He said, "PTSD gets into every part of the brain." This patient, who had never used clay before, found a remarkable ability to sculpt. He noted that the time allowed him a respite from ongoing intrusive thoughts.

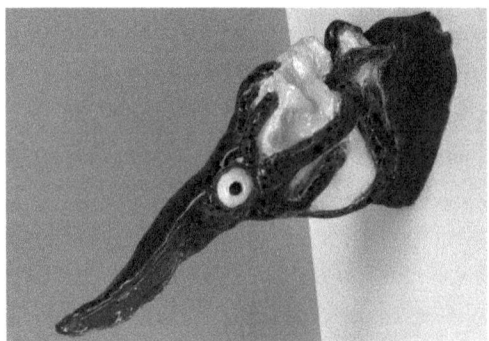

Figure 7.1: A service member's self-portrait

The secondary reward in the clay hand building is the glazing application. Patients brush dull substances over their pieces without a clear vision of what it will look like after firing. This parallels with letting go of the controls anxiety produces, and facilitates the mantra "Trust the process." After pieces are returned glossy and colorful from the final fire, the service members find instant gratification. Conversations abound with their peers about what glazes and techniques were used. This motivates others to work and find the same delight.

THE MILITARY GROUP ART THERAPIST'S SKILL SET

It cannot be ignored that my varied art therapy experience with groups and individuals has been extremely valuable in working within the active-duty population. For the most part, the service members are highly committed to their treatment; however, what brought them to this point ranges from a single trauma event to issues that have been stacking up against them since early childhood. Examples include child abuse, abandonment, poverty, neurobehavioral disorders, learning disabilities, substance abuse, marital conflict, and borderline and other psychiatric disorders. The list goes on. Some expect to separate from military service after hospital treatment, and others return to work. Some patients continue treatment part-time on a hospital program and a small percentage are transferred to another inpatient program. Whatever their outcome, the service member is used to being trained and expects a high level of competency from the therapist. For art therapists, knowing media, their properties and endless applications distinguishes them from the therapist who may incorporate art directives in talk therapy groups. Service members come to me with a vision and want assistance as to how to execute the process. Guiding individuals through their process helps to establish trust and sense of safety. I juggle these expectations by imparting my art therapy goals and how they differ from the art education perspective that is most familiar. By patients being assisted to focus on the process and not the product, insights are gained as they recognize how their internal talk and external relationships are mirrored in this therapy.

To meet the needs of the masses, being organized and open to maintaining a plethora of art supplies, craft items, and recycled materials is advised. Having that special item—be it a dowel rod, a hinge, fabric paint, glitter, a scrap of leather—provides the patient with endless possibilities to unleash that long withheld creative energy. Being competent with multicultural and LBGTQ (lesbian, bisexual, gay, transgender and questioning) areas enables the art therapist to aid individuals exploring issues that have impacted their emotional health. Art facilitates this self-exploration and strengths training. Grief and loss, family systems, and anger management are other reoccurring themes the art therapist needs to be well versed in and ready to tackle. Yalom's (2005) 11 therapeutic factors that influence change and healing in groups are readily seen in art therapy groups. Within the context of art making, service members find universal themes, ways to help one another work together to increase bonding, and see their art as expressions of something bigger than itself. A therapist needs to be proficient in utilizing these factors to maintain a healthy group. Finally, the use of humor and music creates a climate of accessibility and comfort.

CONCLUDING REMARKS

The art therapist must rely on supportive staff. As in any healthy relationship, it takes work, time, and compromise. Staff training in art therapy should be ongoing, whether it is in a formal or informal format. I provide a handout to attending mental health workers that defines art therapy, my intent, ways to help (e.g., safety is a priority) and behaviors to avoid. For example, staff must be educated that art therapy demands the same social distance as other psychotherapy groups. It is natural to look, compliment, and engage in a conversation while a patient is engaged in an art process. A staff member may say, "Oh, I could never do this. I am not creative." These interruptions would be unheard of in a talk therapy group. I remind the co-worker that art making is a prime opportunity to practice mindfulness or experience what Mihaly Csikszentmihalyi (2017) is most noted for: "a state of flow." Additionally, complimenting one patient distracts peers and redirects them to look at their own work critically. It is the art therapist's responsibility to protect the patient by maintaining ethics in regard to how the art is handled, and to educate the treatment team. An employee's compliment may seem harmless, as may a request to a skillful patient to paint them a picture for their home. Though it is acceptable for a patient to give their art to whomever they wish, I generally discourage this. More often, our patients leave art for incoming patients to see. Those in treatment for combat trauma will leave a compelling piece to display in a designated group room where they share their war stories. These walls are overwhelming evidence of the impact of trauma that words can hardly express (Furman, 2013).

Though my schedule is not structured for individual therapy, the patient's assigned therapists may seek my guidance if they feel the patient will progress using art in their course of individualized treatment. I may meet with the service member for a few sessions or simply counsel briefly and provide supplies so they can do the work on their own. A service member may approach me with an assignment such as "My therapist wants me to make art about my strengths." We then look for methods and media that the patient can find meaningful and engaging. Sometimes, individual art therapy is arranged in cases of severely depressed patients or with comorbid conditions such as traumatic brain injury who are unable to see change through talk therapies.

Honoring the work of individuals is another layer of therapeutic value. This may be a simple act of coating acrylic paintings with a shellac to enrich the surface, matting a special watercolor and drawing in order to have it displayed at the patient's home. Clay works that cannot be transported in the service members' luggage are carefully wrapped, packaged, and mailed to their stated destination. I have been told by patients over the course of time who may have had to return to treatment, "Yes, I got my package. Thank you so much for mailing it to me." When they share this news with their peers, it seems to communicate trust and a care for them as an individual. It also helps many relax and be open to make stuff as the worry of "How am I going to get it home?"

is easily resolved. The calendar mentioned early on is distributed to the public and sent to all the contributors and their families if designated. This has given a voice to our patients and helps to lower the stigma of having treatment.

Aftercare creative arts resources are made available to the patients for continuum of care. This may include finding art therapists, art supply retail stores, and art community groups in the area the service members are to return to. I provide a list of the supplies on request that I use in my art directives. Service members often ask for a supply list because they want to do art with their children when they get home. We talk about age-appropriate activities for their children, ways to encourage creative expression, and adaptations for those with special needs. Some of the workshops I facilitated on our Joint Base San Antonio Medical Center Caregiver Support Program for Wounded Warriors included art that represented self-care, family trees, and safe environments. Spouses and children were able to express their challenges and needs safely through the power of their imagery. It is clear that a need exists to develop more art therapy resources for the families and caregivers of our veterans.

In closing, this chapter was intended to lay a groundwork of ideas and approaches to working with large art therapy inpatient active-duty groups. I have avoided sharing personal anecdotes because I would not be able to give them their due justice in the context of this chapter. Also, I feel that it would be a dishonor to the individuals who gave me their permission while in treatment to open that vulnerable part of them that had been so stoutly guarded and locked away. That is their story not mine; I am simply the catalyst that helps put the stories into art forms for healing and sharing through the power of the group.

Chapter 8

Art Therapy in an Active-Duty Military Substance Abuse Rehabilitation Clinic

COURTNEY BENNETT AND KEVIN D'AUGUSTINE

INTRODUCTION

The following is informed by the work of the two authors as art therapists at a military substance abuse rehabilitation clinic in Virginia serving active-duty service members of all four branches. The first author is a licensed professional counselor and registered art therapist who has served as the full-time art therapist for the program for over two years. In addition to working with active-duty military in the clinic, she was part of the military culture as a dependent. Her husband spent six years in the U.S. Army. The second author served ten years in the U.S. military prior to becoming an art therapist. Since graduating from an art therapy graduate program, he has worked in multiple military mental health clinics and spends 75 percent of his time in the substance abuse rehabilitation clinic.

Over the course of their work in the clinic, the authors have created, modified, and implemented many art therapy directives and experientials for use with the patient population to support the established recovery goals of the clinic and enable patient personal development. This chapter will provide an overview of art therapy directives and experientials, how art therapy supports the clinic's and patients' goals, and some observations of patient responses to art therapy within the substance abuse rehabilitation milieu.

Art therapy is lauded within this particular substance abuse rehabilitation clinic. Lewis, Dana, and Blevins (2015) espoused that "substance counseling requires a fresh approach, a new mindset, and, in fact, a new definition" (p.15) and that it should be complex and collaborative. The leadership of the clinic subscribes to the same thinking and thoroughly supports a multi-faceted approach to rehabilitation. Both military and civilian staff are enthusiastic in their support of art therapy and other therapies that augment the traditional discussion group format.

THE PROGRAM

The more intense treatment levels addressed in this chapter are the intensive outpatient (IOP) and inpatient levels, also referred to as levels 2 and 3, respectively. The patients in the two levels progress through the program together, with the only differences between the groups being that the IOP patients leave the building at the end of the treatment day, are responsible for getting to Alcoholics Anonymous (AA) or Narcotics Anonymous (NA) meetings on their own in the evenings, and are subject to mandatory drug/alcohol screenings at the start of every treatment week.

The program for levels 2 and 3 is composed of a five-week schedule of small group discussions, workshops, assignments, AA and NA meetings, mental health counseling sessions, medication interventions (as needed), recreation therapy sessions, and art therapy sessions. The level to which a patient is assigned is determined by their command's recommendation, the service member's living situation, safety concerns, the likelihood of the patient being tempted by and obtaining substances, and the severity of detoxification at entry. A patient can be moved from one level to another depending on the same factors plus their participation, attitude, and rule adherence.

REFERRALS

A service member can self-refer to the program or be referred by their command. Command referrals far outnumber self-referrals. Among the self-referrals are the true self-referrals, as well as those who are "highly encouraged" by their commands to self-refer. The latter situation is referred to as being "volun-told." Self-referring reflects better on a service member, suggesting that they have identified an area in need of improvement and are being proactive. A command referral is typically initiated by an alcohol-related incident (ARI), a punishable offense in which alcohol is likely a contributing factor. Examples of common ARIs include driving under the influence/driving while impaired (DUI/DWI) offenses, physical altercations, domestic violence, property damage, public intoxication, and self-injurious behavior or suicide attempts. ARIs are sometimes the first indicators that alert commands to a service member's problem with substances. Other indicators include a service member missing work, reporting to work late due to substance use, reporting to work intoxicated or high, or "popping positive" on a urinalysis. Urinalysis testing is done frequently in military services; commands hold random urinalysis screenings for their personnel, but service members can also be selected for screening if they are even suspected of drug use or intoxication while on duty.

Command responses to alcohol-related incidents can vary. U.S. Department of the Navy (2009) regulations state:

Commanders, commanding officers, and Officers in Charge (OICs) must exercise sound judgment in enforcing Navy's alcohol and drug abuse policies and ensure proper disposition of individual cases. They must analyse all available evidence to determine whether alcohol or drug abuse exists and shall respond to unacceptable behavior or substandard performance with appropriate corrective actions. (U.S. Department of the Navy, 2009)

The other military branches have similar wording in their regulations. Some commands are stricter than others, irrespective of a service member's performance, attitude, and personality. Other commands factor in those things when deciding the level of rehabilitation needed and their disposition (retention or discharge from service) after completion of a rehab program. Service members often know what awaits them after finishing the program, but not always. Of major concern for the service members is their future following completion of the program. Some know in advance of attending the program whether they face discharge from service in the near future. Others discover their fate while in treatment. Service regulations, the command's attitude towards the service member, and the nature of an offense all combine to help determine the disposition of the service member. Some not only face discharge, but also civilian or military legal action, including incarceration. Some are seen as just needing a little help with rehabilitation and are expected back at their commands after treatment.

Many factors can influence a service member's attitude towards treatment, including referral type (command referral or self-referral), level of treatment (intensive outpatient or inpatient), separation from family, potential legal issues (including post-treatment incarceration), potential discharge, disagreement with a substance use diagnosis, co-occurring mood or personality disorders, and interpersonal issues within the inpatient community.

Potential outcomes include retention or discharge from service, with or without punitive measures. A service member's attitude towards their immediate future is determined by whether or not their post-treatment disposition aligns with their desire to stay in or leave the military. As expected, attitudes towards their military service, command, and rehabilitation can be greatly affected by knowing or not knowing what will happen following completion of the program. As one can imagine, anxiety levels among the population can be quite high at times. These anxieties are significant factors in a patient's attitude when coming into the art room. Common contributors to high anxiety include low self-esteem, discomfort in social situations, extreme depression, fear of failure, and fear of judgment. Other major factors that have been seen to affect patient attitude towards art making include past art-making experiences, attitudes of defiance, traumatic brain injury, developmental delays, substance-related cognitive impairments, and disbelief in the efficacy of non-traditional treatments in substance abuse recovery.

ART THERAPY GROUPS

Every week, a new cohort of patients—a mix of level 2s and level 3s—arrives at the clinic to begin treatment. The cohort size varies, typically between 8 and 16 patients. The program consists of one week of on-boarding and familiarization classes, called "INDOC," after which new patients enter the general population. During INDOC week, members of each new cohort are assigned a small discussion group, identified by a color (e.g., "Group Orange"). The discussion groups are supported by multiple addictions counselors and a mental health counselor (a PsyD or LCSW). Assigning new patients to different groups ensures that the various groups get an influx of new participants, therefore keeping the groups full of patients in different weeks of treatment. This allows senior patients to model behaviors, share knowledge, demonstrate growth, and exemplify the recovery process to newer patients. Patients are identified by their group names for administrative purposes and certain treatment considerations, but they are also identified by their week of treatment. The week identifiers allow them to move with their cohort through weekly workshops, recreation therapy groups, and art therapy groups, allowing those offerings to focus on goals identified as appropriate for patients of a treatment week.

In regard to art therapy groups, patients are seen both as weekly cohorts and as groups identified by their group name. Art therapy directives for the different weeks generally support the treatment goals established for those weeks. As in most settings, when first meeting patients, it is important to build rapport. This begins during INDOC week. In their first art therapy group, patients are introduced to the studio, materials, art therapists, and art therapy as a treatment modality.

The directives provided during week one address identity and develop communication skills. The second week of treatment focuses on identifying emotions, developing an emotions-wise vocabulary, and understanding the degree to which they can be tolerated and expressed. Week three focuses on the patients identifying resources of strength and resiliency, developing mindfulness practices, and developing personal concept. In week four of treatment, the directives focus on reflection of personal growth, future growth, and established resources. These are general targets considered when selecting a directive for any art therapy session, but other considerations include the needs of the individuals in the group, group energy, recent events in the facility, group size, group anxiety levels, and so on.

In addition to the art therapy sessions offered to the weekly cohorts, the small discussion groups take part in a mask-making session approximately once a month, the goals of which are described below in the directive descriptions. The addictions counselors for the discussion groups are invited into the art room for the verbal processing. Because the group counselors best know their patients' histories, struggles, and personalities, their participation in the verbal processing tends to be very productive. The art therapist and addiction counselors' joint engagement of patients from complementary therapeutic angles is unique and valuable. The addiction counselors often comment on the added value of the mask groups to the therapeutic milieu, particularly in encouraging patients to process their personal narrative, reflect on traumas, and share with others.

Some frequently used art directives are explained below. Each description includes when the directive is typically used, objectives, goals, materials, procedures, and observed outcomes. In addition to the directives detailed below, other directives are frequently offered as workshops, including plaster hand making, paper marbling, string painting (with and without projection), printmaking, intuitive painting, container making projects, and other standard art therapy directives geared towards individual and group communication, growth, affect regulation, trauma processing, and so on. Some directives are chosen to probe and push patients towards a deeper understanding, while others are provided as a means of self-expression, as a creative outlet, or as a much-needed break from talking. Regardless of the overt purpose of an art therapy group, in the substance abuse rehabilitation environment, as in so many others, in the words of Natalie Rogers (2001, p.163), "What is creative is often therapeutic."

DIRECTIVES
SELF-ADVERTISEMENT: WEEK 1
Objective: This directive explores the role of self-esteem in developing identity and self-concept. The objective is to support the patients' ability to explore identity and identify desired and undesired attributes.

Goals:

- Communicate personal characteristics and values to others
- Practice assertive communication
- Develop self-esteem
- Introduce group members and build rapport

Materials:

- Magazines
- Collage materials
- Drawing materials (pastels, markers, pencils, etc.)
- India inks
- Scissors
- Glue

Procedure: 1 hour, 15 minutes (55 minutes art process, 20 minutes processing). Time varies depending on number of group members.

Open the group with a discussion about the purpose of advertising for products on TV and in magazines. Ask patients about the purpose of advertisements, assisting them if necessary, to identify the goal of selling something by showing off the best qualities of that product. Ask patients to imagine they have to "sell" themselves in an advertisement and to think about what qualities they would most want to show off to others. Invite patients to create their advertisement using materials of their choice.

With about 15 minutes remaining in the art-making process, the art therapist can ask patients to include a disclaimer in the advertisement. This can be a "warning or side effect" of which the patients are aware and which they would like to improve on while in treatment. It is important to not introduce this aspect too early, because some patients may focus more on this negative element and avoid identifying their positive traits.

Typical outcomes/observations: This is usually the first group together and some patients may be hesitant about drawing, which is why it is important to include collage materials. The India inks are also a nice way to begin a process, allowing patients to simply get color on the page.

This specific directive provides insight for the art therapist, allowing them to get a feel for a patient's established, or lack of established, identity. Patients will sometimes struggle with the idea of identity because they cannot remember what a sober identity looks like for them. The directive can also provide data regarding the patient's self-worth and possible ambivalence towards their sobriety.

Patients who struggle with approaching the process are encouraged to use the India inks to allow them to begin the process. The looseness of the inks sometimes helps patients become more comfortable and inspires them to add to the advertisement using other materials. The spontaneity and abstraction of the materials can also serve as a metaphor for a patient's identity.

POSTCARD: WEEK 1

Objective: Through this process, patients can explore their current understanding of recovery, future goals, and find inspiration with which to reach their goals.

Goals:

- Identify personal qualities and characteristics
- Identify areas for change/improvement
- Develop communication skills
- Build rapport

Materials:

- Paper (6″ x 9″)
- Drawing materials (pastels, markers, pencils, etc.)
- India inks

Procedure: 1 hour, 15 minutes (55 minutes art process, 20 minutes processing). Time varies depending on number of group members.

"Create a postcard to your future self at week 4 of treatment. Write about what you hope to work on while in treatment, goals, what you hope to get out of your experiences, and so on. On the other side of the postcard, create art in response to your writing. (This can be a symbol of hope for the future.)"

A great way to start this process is with bullet journaling. Allow the patients about five minutes to write anything and everything that is on their mind. This can help clear their minds and allow them to focus on the directive presented.

Typical outcomes/observations: This directive is typically introduced to a group of patients who have expressed interest in writing as a way to process, reflect, or ground themselves. There have been mixed responses when using this directive. Many patients who are serious about their sobriety will invest time in the message that they write to themselves, whereas patients who may be ambivalent about treatment often show more defenses in their writing reflection and art response.

EMOTIONS IDENTIFICATION: WEEK 2

Objective: Through this directive, patients can expand their understanding of emotions, strengthen emotional vocabulary, increase awareness of similarities and differences in processing of emotions, and regulate anxiety.

Goals:

- Strengthen vocabulary as it relates to emotions
- Recognize complexities and nuances of different emotions
- Recognize similarities and differences between people when expressing emotions

Materials:

For Part 1:

- 3″ x 5″ pieces of drawing paper (see procedure for quantity)
- Oil and chalk pastels

For Part 2:

- Handouts with large list of emotions (one per patient)

For Part 3:

- Set of cards (eight or more) with one emotion written on each
- A list or word bank with all the emotions included in this card set

Procedure:

Part 1: Compare and contrast

This part consists of patients making small drawings for a set of emotions, then comparing and contrasting the artwork they make. Small cards (3″ x 5″) are recommended. Prior to the session, create a set of cards consisting of at least the number of patients you will have. On each, write a different emotion and a big "X" on one side. Repeat until you have several identical stacks of cards with the same emotions in the same order.

Explain that expressive or abstract art is preferred when depicting the emotions graphically. If necessary, explain what expressive and abstract art are and what they are not. The goal is to express an abstract concept (an emotion) and to avoid depicting people (or stick figures) doing things, facial expressions, and recognizable symbols.

Distribute one set of the emotion cards among the patients. Ask patients to think about the emotion written on their card, a time when they experienced the emotion, and to depict it graphically using shapes, lines, and colors. Instruct patients to draw on the side opposite the written emotion and a big "X". Give them three minutes to do this, then collect the cards. Repeat with a second set of cards, distributing them so that patients do not receive the same emotion a second time. Collect those cards after three minutes. Repeat the process for each remaining set of cards. If all card sets are in the same order, the therapist can simply start distribution at a different starting point with each set to ensure no one gets the same emotion more than once.

While patients are drawing, the therapist can be taping the emotions cards on a wall or whiteboard, grouping the emotions into columns. At the end of all the card sets, ask patients to put away their materials while the last set is added to the wall. The therapist should now have several columns of cards taped up, one per emotion. The therapist can now ask patients to compare and contrast the different images in a column. For example: "What are some similarities you see in the 'anger' column? What differences?" It is hoped that patients will be able to identify colors and formal elements of art that appear to be more common. Likewise, they should be able to identify any unique elements.

Note: The "compare and contrast" part is an opportunity for the therapist to point out that we experience and process some emotions similarly, but that individual experiences and personality can make our responses unique. Additionally, point out that cultural differences may exist in the understanding or expression of emotions. *The discussion can lead to how humans express emotions physiologically—there may be similarities between many people in how their anger presents, but there are also some differences. Example: it may be easy to identify someone getting red-faced, balling their fists, or glaring as experiencing anger. But, conversely, some people internalize, disconnect, and stew quietly. We can take cues from body language, but keep in mind the importance of verbal communication when dealing with emotions. Assumptions can lead to misunderstandings.*

Part 2: Emotions list

Prior to the session, obtain or create a large list of emotions. There should be many in workbooks and on the internet from which to choose. Make photocopies of this list available to each patient. Ask patients to go through the list and mark each emotion they have experienced since being in the rehabilitation program. Give several minutes for this, then ask them to identify one of the emotions they have felt the most intensely. Ask for volunteers to share the situations that triggered the emotion.

This part provides a chance to confront the patients who claim not to have emotions. The therapist can point out how many they have marked on their list. The therapist can also poll the group when stories are shared, asking if anyone else has experienced the same situations or emotions and how they handled them.

Part 3: Charades

Post a list or word bank of emotions which matches the emotions written on the set of charades cards.

Hold cards out (or spread cards out on a table) for volunteers to select, one at a time. Invite the patient to "set the scene," using words if necessary, then act out the emotion for the other patients to guess. Patients guessing can use the emotions word bank to help narrow down which emotion the actor is portraying. Members of the audience can call out the emotion they believe is being portrayed until the correct one is given. The actor will acknowledge when the correct emotion is stated. Repeat as time allows.

This part allows for anxiety reduction and emotional discharge. This is sometimes a good opportunity to point out how some emotions can be portrayed in similar ways. For example, one person's embarrassment may appear like someone else's rejection.

Typical outcomes/observations: These groups are typically limited to no more than eight patients. The vibe of this group has been very diverse, ranging from nearly an entire group taking part enthusiastically, to one patient being resistant and minimally engaged, to several people exhibiting minimal investment or interest. Often, the resistant patients are guarded and hesitant to even express their emotions graphically, and some have even challenged the therapeutic value of such a directive.

Of all the difficulties that arise during this directive, the most prevalent is the patients' use of representational depictions of emotions—stick figures with expressions on their faces, stick figures in recognizable situations, tears, sunrises, and so on. Despite being shown a graphic spectrum of artistic styles and reiterating that abstract and expressionist depictions are preferred, some patients still tend towards more symbolic and representational art.

Another phenomenon often encountered is the occurrence of some patients making art on the same side of the paper as the written emotion. Doing so affects the next step of guessing the emotions by graphic elements only (it is not hard to guess the emotion when it is written above the image). We found that placing a large "X" over the side with the written emotion prevents the issue.

CREATE–DESTROY–CREATE: WEEK 2

Objective: This process allows patients to identify emotions with which they struggle, to reflect on them, and to physically/mentally transform them into something new. This process allows for a shift in thinking, understanding, and emotional regulation.

Goals:

- Recognize tendencies to avoid specific emotions
- Recognize tendencies to seek out experiencing specific emotions
- Develop emotional language to process emotions
- Identify coping skills

Materials:

- Drawing materials (pastels, markers, pencils, etc.)
- Paper, medium (about 9″ x 12″) and large (about 12″ x 18″)
- Glue sticks

Procedure: 1 hour, 15 minutes (55 minutes art process, 20 minutes processing). Time varies depending on number of group members.

Patients are asked to identify one or more "negative" emotions they have felt since being in the rehabilitation clinic and to depict it/them graphically on a medium-sized piece of paper. Urge patients to be expressive with shapes, lines, and color. After allowing 15–20 minutes, lead a discussion, asking patients to share about an emotion they identified and a situation that provoked the emotion. Ask the group about shared experiences and triggers.

At a comfortable point in the discussion, ask the patients to rip, cut, or otherwise destroy the artwork that they made. Expect hesitance from some and excitement from others. Reiterate that there is a reason for this, which will become clearer at the end of the session. As patients are destroying their artwork, distribute the large pieces of paper. Ask patients to use tape, glue, or use some other method to incorporate pieces of their destroyed artwork into a new artwork reflecting a "positive" emotion. The "positive" emotion can be either one they have experienced while in the program or one they hope to experience again during recovery.

After approximately 20–30 minutes, begin a discussion on what the experience was like for patients, focusing on the difficulty they may have had destroying their first piece of art. Discussion can flush out why it was difficult for some, identifying if it was the aversion to destroying something they spent time making, aversion to destroying a piece of art they liked, or being comfortable sitting with the "negative" emotion. Explain that people often prefer what they know, even if it is uncomfortable, and discuss patients' hesitance to give up an emotion they have experienced for a long time. Conversely, discuss positive feelings related to the destruction and transformation of the first artwork into the second one.

Typical outcomes/observations: As stated above, some patients will hesitate to destroy their first piece of artwork depicting a "negative" emotion. Some patients have chosen not to cut or rip their artwork, but to fold or crumple it instead. On occasion, a patient will simply rip a small piece out of a corner. Recreating the artwork has also been seen in which patients used glue or tape to reconstruct the image like a puzzle, securing it to the larger sheet of paper. Many times, reassurance is needed for patients to trust the process. The hesitation in destroying their artwork allows for questions to be asked, like, "Why was it difficult to destroy the negative emotion?" Many times, patients have become used to feeling this emotion or it is a better-known and more understood emotion than "positive" emotions. Once the patients are able to create the second image, they usually respond by feeling better and more relaxed, but not always.

DEPICT YOURSELF AS A TREE: WEEK 2

Objectives: This process allows patients to reflect on their strengths and areas in which they desire improvement/change.

Goals:

- Identify strengths
- Identify areas for improvement/change

Materials:

- Drawing materials (pastels, markers, pencils, etc.)
- Paper, white (12" x 18")
- Collage papers (construction paper, tissue paper, foils, etc.)
- Scissors
- Glue sticks

Procedure: 1 hour, 15 minutes (55 minutes art process, 20 minutes processing). Time varies depending on number of group members.

Ask patients to think of themselves as a tree. Invite them to reflect on the roots as a tree's strength and to make correlations with their strengths, thinking about morals, values, and other attributes. Then ask patients to consider the leaves of the tree as those things that are shed and equate them to unwanted behaviors and elements in their lives. Ask patients to use the materials to depict themselves as a tree, writing their strengths in the roots and their unwanted aspects in the leaves. Discuss this with them.

Typical outcomes/observations: This directive allows for reflection and insight into the patients' strengths and motivation for sobriety. This tree directive also allows for the formal elements of art therapy to be observed. Developmental age, depression, and anxiety may surface through the patients' artwork and process.

RECOVERY ISLAND: WEEK 3

Objective: Art therapy can be a great practice when working with peers to identify needs in recovery. It can also assist in finding the individuality and advocacy a patient may need when around their peers, family, and friends. During recovery, patients will need to identify the differences between want and need and why it is important to do so.

Goals:

- Identify personal values
- Identify resources
- Identify strengths and weaknesses
- Identify wants and needs
- Practice communication skills and advocating for oneself

Materials:

- Paper, large (20" x 30" or greater) or poster board (one per pair or small group)
- Drawing materials (pastels, markers, pencils, etc.)

Procedure: 1 hour, 15 minutes (55 minutes art process, 20 minutes processing). Time varies depending on number of group members.

Patients work in pairs or small groups, depending on the group size. Direct patients to create a private island that would be the perfect, ideal world in which to live. Encourage patients to identify who they would want on the island, what resources they believe they would need to survive on the island, what defenses they would need, what activities they would want, the possibility of leaving the island, and how they might feel in such a place. Share and process drawings afterwards. With about five minutes remaining in the art-making part, ask patients to think of a name for their island.

Typical outcomes/observations: It is interesting to take note of who includes a bar or club on their island. Some patients have included depictions of alcohol bottles, joints, and pot leaves. Most often, when questioned about their reasoning for including substances in their perfect world, patients reply that in their "perfect, ideal world" they do not have a problem with alcohol or other substances and can partake responsibly. Also, frequently seen are churches or other buildings specifically for AA or NA meetings. The therapist can discuss group cohesion and inclusion, communication styles, comfort working in the small groups, self-advocacy, appropriateness in the design process and depiction of resources, and so on.

▓ ROAD MAP TO RECOVERY: WEEK 3

Objective: Art therapists can help point out things patients might not have noticed during sessions in order to stimulate critical thinking and insight. Patients can use art for relaxation, as a coping skill, to solve problems, and to practice communication. This group identifies the struggles and milestones of the recovery journey.

Goals:

- Identify potential challenges of recovery
- Identify coping skills and response behaviors to unforeseen challenges
- Recognize resources and support systems

Materials:

- Paper, large (~12" x 18")
- Drawing materials (pastels, markers, pencils, etc.)
- Paint
- Brushes
- Collage materials
- Scissors
- Glue

Procedure: 1 hour, 15 minutes (55 minutes art process, 20 minutes processing). Time varies depending on number of group members.

Ask patients to use drawing and/or collage materials to depict a road running from the rehabilitation clinic to some point in the future. Encourage patients to select a realistic goal in the future, such as one year of sobriety, discharging from the military, re-enlisting, seeing their families, moving house. Ask patients to think about the metaphor of a road and to depict how they foresee their path after completing rehabilitation on their way to their goal. Remind patients of the types of things seen on road trips, such as gas stations, rest areas, detours, varying terrain, obstacles, different road conditions, and to use those items to reflect on the supports, resources, obstacles, difficulties, and triggers they may experience in real life as they approach their goal. Discuss as a group.

Typical outcomes/observations: Sometimes a patient will depict a road with no obstacles or resources. When questioned, patients who do this explain that there is no way to know what the future holds. Some identify their sobriety and new attitude as that which will get them through whatever life may throw at them; others just cannot envision how their futures may look. This process allows patients to reflect on what they still need out of their treatment while in the program. During this session, patients are sometimes able to identify previously unforeseen needs, which they can bring up during the interdisciplinary treatment team meeting that occurs during their third week of treatment.

TRANSITIONAL OBJECT (RECOVERY COIN): WEEK 4

Objectives: Art therapy can serve as a process to foster resiliency in patients. The transitional object can be something they are taking away from the patient experience in treatment. This can serve as a reminder of what they are working towards, what they have overcome, or serve as a source of grounding.

Goals:

- Encourage reflection
- Identify resources of strength
- Promote resiliency

Materials:

- Shrinky Dinks® material
- Permanent markers, Sharpies®
- Colored pencils
- Hole punch

Procedure: 30–60 minutes. (Because this group was scheduled for the last full day of treatment, patients were released when they were done working to prepare for discharge. No processing was conducted.)

Patients are introduced to Shrinky Dinks® material and shown examples of finished "coins." Ask patients to explore what they want to take away from their experience in the rehabilitation clinic. This can be words of encouragement, a reminder of what they are working towards, things they have overcome, an object on which to focus and stay present, and so on. Reviewing the instructions on Shrinky Dinks® packaging, the therapist should instruct patients on which materials work best on the plastic material. A handout with the instructions can be provided in the event that patients would like to repeat the process in the future. The handout can have several outlines of circles in which to brainstorm designs for a "coin."

When ready, a Shrinky Dinks® plastic sheet with a pre-drawn circle, the same size as the one on the handout, is given to the patient. Patients then trace the design onto the plastic. It is difficult to erase from this material, so it is important to encourage patients to create a draft of their design on paper first. Once they have completed the design on the plastic, they cut out the circle. Shrinking the coins can be done in a toaster oven or conventional oven. Follow the instructions on the Shrinky Dinks® packaging.

The recovery coin instructions and practice sheet is provided below.

Typical outcomes/observations: This process is one of the directives most anticipated by the patients. If possible, it is best to be able to shrink the coins while in session. More can be discussed about seeing the coin shrink. During the shrinking process, the material tends to become distorted and then returns to its circular, flat shape. This can parallel a patient's journey to treatment or towards sobriety.

RECOVERY COIN INSTRUCTIONS AND DESIGN SHEET

A *transitional object* is something that can be used during times of change to focus attention and remind you of where you've been and where you are going. In your last week of treatment, you are given the opportunity to create a recovery coin, which you design, to remind you of your goals and your progress. Some people choose to put a phrase, words of encouragement, reminders, or images on their coin. You can use the circles below to work on your design idea. When you are satisfied with it, you can trace it on to the Shrinky Dinks® plastic sheet, which, when heated by the art therapist, will shrink down to about 1.5 inches in diameter. Notice there is a smooth side and a rough side to the plastic.

Art making tips:

1. Sharpies® work well on both sides. Pencils, color pencils, and markers only work on the rough side.
2. Colors become more intense when the coin is shrunk.
3. Do not write too small. Letters shrink and will be hard to read if too small.
4. Do not make artwork too detailed. Details may be lost when shrunk.
5. If you'd like to make a key ring, holes must be punched (two holes close together, like a figure "8") and not too close to the edge. (Art therapists have hole punches.)
6. When your design is drawn on the plastic, cut out the circle and give it to an art therapist to shrink.

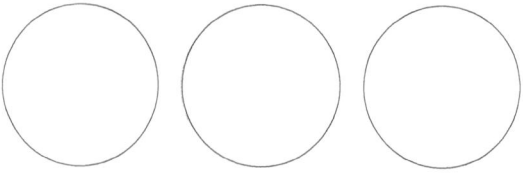

Good luck to you on your journey. You can use your coin as a reminder of the progress you are making towards your goals and your successful completion of the rehabilitation program.

MASK-MAKING

Note: Patients attend this group at least once while in treatment. This group is typically offered on a monthly rotation basis to the small discussion groups.

Objective: This art therapy process focuses on exploring personal identity, assesses the impact of substances on decision-making, and recognizes the impact of past behaviors on present functioning. This art process allows patients to explore layers of identity that are usually hidden and not shared with others. It is an opportunity to identify these areas visually and create a metaphor to explore difficult topics. The art therapy process can assist in finding the vocabulary to verbally share their process.

Goals:

- Identify private and public emotions
- Identify personal characteristics
- Develop healthy boundaries
- Practice assertiveness skills

Materials:

- Face-shaped mask for each patient
- Acrylic and/or watercolor paints
- Drawing materials (pastels, markers, pencils, etc.)
- Scissors
- Glue/Mod Podge®
- Magazines
- Collage materials (feathers, sequins, tissue paper, etc.)
- Model Magic®

Procedure: 2 hours, 30 minutes (1.5 hours art process, 1 hour verbal processing).

The group begins with a discussion about masks and how they have served humans throughout history in a variety of ways: to entertain, to frighten, to go to war, to hide aspects, or for anonymity. The concept of personas can be briefly discussed. The most recognized opportunities to wear different metaphorical masks (personas) are identified as work life and home life. Patients are encouraged to discuss the differences in what they hide and what they show in both environments. Patients are asked if they feel that these masks ever come off completely. This can move into discussion of how we may layer our masks, but if we never take the time to take them off, substances may come into play.

Patients are asked to remove their metaphoric masks and look inside at the things they are hiding or avoiding and then display them visually on the paper mask. We encourage patients to invest all they can into the art process, keeping in mind that during verbal discussion they can decide how much to disclose verbally. In this way, patients are encouraged to express everything, while allowing them to control their disclosures at their level of comfort.

Note: In this clinic, the small-group addiction counselors are invited in for the verbal processing part. It is beneficial for art therapists to establish themselves as the facilitator of the discussion and for the counselors to understand that they are welcome to take part in the dialogue when cued by the art therapist. The inclusion of the addictions counselors in the verbal processing is very useful due to their deeper knowledge of the patients' personal histories, goals, and personalities. In this environment, it has been seen that in working together, the art therapist and the addictions counselors can help the patients move into new emotional territory and understanding that endure and expand their small-group discussions.

Typical outcomes/observations: It is interesting to note that, on the few occasions when the mask-making groups are temporarily halted, both small-group counselors and patients express disappointment. The counselors also regularly express their appreciation for the sessions because they frequently get to patient issues that were repressed, denied, or difficult to tease out through discussion alone. This supports Wilson's (2001, p.49) claim that "it is common for patients to readily speak about the story or meaning of their art productions, after maintaining a stony silence when offered the opportunity simply to speak about themselves and their problems."

As a testament to the emotional power of this directive, patients have found themselves in deeper or unexpected levels of self-reflection and have been compelled to face certain issues. As Rubin (2001, p.18) points out: "The shock of discovering previously unknown and usually unwanted aspects of the self is often visceral. The excitement of not only seeing—but also feeling—connections between what has been known and what has been hidden is equally powerful." The heightened sensitivity that sometimes arises from making a mask has, at times, warranted a patient being placed on the "high interest" list for increased safety checks. Some patients have even voluntarily self-discharged from the program against medical advice following a mask-making group. In those situations, the art making was just one of multiple contributing factors influencing patient decisions, but it remains a potent element within the addictions rehabilitation milieu. Strong emotions can be activated in patients during this directive, and counselors and therapists should continue to monitor patients closely if concerns arise.

▓ WORKSHOP: SEEKING SAFETY

Objective: Art therapy uses a variety of expressive materials and processes to help patients explore thoughts and emotions in a creative, nonthreatening way. Mindfulness practices through art making can provide focus and grounding, and create a safe environment for reflection.

Goals:

- Identify resources for strength and resiliency
- Develop personal self-concept
- Explore intrapersonal relationships
- Establish healthy boundaries and trust in interpersonal relationships
- Develop grounding techniques for self-soothing

Materials:

- Canvas
- Acrylic paints
- Paintbrushes
- Drawing materials (pastels, markers, pencils, etc.)

Procedure: Ask patients to paint an image of something that makes them feel safe, such as a specific place, person, or symbol. Afterwards, ask patients to share their work and discuss issues of trust, authenticity, and relaxation.

Typical outcomes/observations: It is important for patients exploring difficult topics and issues to have a sense of safety. There are many variations in presenting the idea of a safe place and ways it can be created through an art process. One example is presenting a guided imagery meditation that allows the patient to explore their safe place utilizing their senses. Other directives can create a safe place using a box. The outer portion can serve as the defenses protecting the inside, which represents that safe place. This same idea can be depicted using paper and including flaps that can fold over the safe place.

CONCLUSION

Working with active-duty service members in a substance abuse program, as in many other military treatment facilities, provides art therapists with an opportunity to engage with a multi-dimensional culture. One can look at each patient through disparate lenses, focusing on their inherited culture (i.e., ethnicity and upbringing), military culture, and the individual. Military culture is complex, demanding, and sometimes dangerous. It can be the source of pride for many, but also of stress and trauma. The contractual obligation of being in military service can complicate life for those with substance abuse concerns. People cannot just quit their jobs, distance themselves from all bad influences, take a mental health day, and seek support in complete anonymity. Stigma is a serious consideration and is even harder to understand within an environment that seemingly encourages alcohol consumption. Service members sometimes receive mixed messages from peers, military history and tradition, and some leaders' tales of drunken adventures, while also receiving safety briefings warning of alcohol abuse, drinking and driving, underage drinking, and no-tolerance drug policies.

The content that surfaces through the art therapy directives can be unique to military life, but the underlying connections to human wants and needs are the same. Under every uniform, the usual human concerns are at the core: lost relationships, traumas, fears of the unknown, change, unhealthy behaviors, shame, guilt, hurt—and sometimes underlying mental health pathologies. The particular directives listed here are not all-inclusive and we reiterate that the needs of the patients ultimately drive just how art making is used within the complex and collaborative environment that is a military substance abuse rehabilitation clinic.

Chapter 9

Countertransference When Working with Military Service Members and Veterans

RACHEL MIMS, MEREDITH MCMACKIN,
GIOIA CHILTON, PETER BUOTTE,
AND KEVIN D'AUGUSTINE

Transference and countertransference are concepts presented when therapists first begin their training. We are told to look out for them as they can inform the therapeutic process. Often, however, after our training, we hear no more about transference and countertransference. As someone who works with military veterans and reads literature about this topic, I (Rachel Mims) surprisingly have never come across any articles addressing countertransference and working with veterans before conducting research for this chapter. Also surprisingly (or perhaps not?), while working on this chapter I was only able to find three sources that discussed countertransference when working with this population.

Galloucis and Kaufman (1988) wrote about group therapy with Vietnam veterans and discussed countertransference from the point of view of a civilian therapist. The authors stated that civilian therapists who lead military or veteran groups are likely to have to "confront feelings within themselves when listening to the details of the provocative actions under-taken by soldiers in a combat zone" (Galloucis & Kaufamn, 1988, p.96);

this statement is true of those working with soldiers from more recent conflicts as well. The authors suggested that therapists should examine the following viewpoints: veterans being either victims or villains, and distress expressed by the veteran is the result of a desire to receive disability compensation. Therapists should also examine their own views about wars, the military, military personnel, and war's impact on a veteran's life.

Melter (2012) conducted a study on the countertransference experiences of psychotherapists who conducted group therapy with combat veterans. Melter identified ten content level themes experienced by the psychotherapists in the study. The first theme identified was "hazing," in that the therapists felt as if the group was bullying them in the initial phase of their group. Questioning the group's value was the second theme that emerged. Facilitators felt as if the group was not benefiting the members; they also struggled with a desire for a different type of group structure than that desired by the group members. This resulted in a struggle for power. Gender was the third theme; male and female facilitators experienced their groups differently, with female therapists reporting more hostility.

In Melter's (2012) study, all therapists were civilians and this fact surfaced in the fourth theme. All of the therapists in the study reported that they felt their group kept them at a distance because of their civilian status. Similarly, the fifth theme was family history of military service. While some groups reacted positively to therapists having a family history of military service, some groups reacted negatively. Along the same lines, theme six was being perceived as an intruder. "This dynamic was often accompanied by an experienced struggle for power or control, and was frequently experienced in conjunction with feelings of isolation or distancing" (Melter, 2012, p.72).

Melter (2012) also found that therapists had experienced a desire to be perceived as "strong" by their group members. All of the therapists "routinely described themselves as inexperienced and as having an incomplete set of clinical skills" (Melter, 2012, p.73). Strong feelings of frustration, fatigue, or exhaustion were experienced by the therapists in the study. They expressed feeling as if they were voyeurs in hearing the veterans' accounts of their combat experiences.

Catherall and Lane (1990) wrote the only article I have found that describes countertransference experienced by therapists who were "vets treating vets." This article talks about the initial bond formed between a therapist who is a veteran and a client who is also a veteran. It states that this bond is formed via shared background and experience, but also that in order to help the client, the therapist will have to rely on a different set of skills from those they relied on when they were in the military. Thus, the therapist is playing both roles: that of warrior (for bonding purposes) and that of therapist (for healing purposes). The authors stated:

> The challenge for the warrior therapist is to be able to maintain the bond that is based on the therapist's warrior identity and still engage the warrior client in the therapeutic tasks of being expressive and vulnerable. The therapist's personal ability to integrate these disparate roles plays an essential part in the development and maintenance of a therapeutic alliance. (Catherall & Lane, 1990, p.24)

Several possible disadvantages to the therapeutic relationship when a veteran treats another veteran were identified by Catherall and Lane (1990); these are things for therapists working with veterans to consider in terms of countertransference. First, along with a possibility for greater understanding comes a possibility for greater misunderstanding if the therapist focuses too much on trauma and not enough on other factors impacting the client's experience. Second, the therapist may lose objectivity due to his or her own personal experiences. Third, the therapist may focus on solutions which worked for him or her and lose focus on the client's strengths. Lastly, exposure to additional trauma via clinical work may re-open the therapist's trauma, resurrect emotional numbing and distancing defenses, and exacerbate survivors' guilt.

Prior to writing this chapter, I had not purposely considered my own countertransference experiences. I have become much more aware of my own reactions to my clients since the idea of this chapter was brought up by another therapist. I have noticed how I really enjoy my interactions with some clients, and how I struggle to stay awake with others! I have noticed that when some clients cancel their appointment I am glad to have the break. Certainly, reading literature about countertransference has opened my eyes beyond what I would have previously identified as a countertransference reaction. While talk therapists use supervision and consultation to deal with countertransference, art therapists also have response art as a method of processing emotions caused by session.

Fish (2019) wrote that art therapists have made response art since the beginning of art therapy. Some art therapists create art after a session and some create art during a session in order to communicate with patients. Kielo (1991) stated that art therapists must not only deal with countertransference related to the client, but also that related to the art. Kielo (1991) reported that post-session artworks were used to develop empathy through replicating a client's image, explore pre-conscious and unconscious, help differentiate affect, explore relationships, and clarify feelings.

While the literature cited in this chapter provides a lot of information on the different ways countertransference can be experienced, it does not provide first-hand accounts of those experiences. I asked several art therapists to write about their own personal experiences with countertransference when working with military service members and/or veterans. The remainder of this chapter contains the four responses that I received. Each individual has provided a short biographical description in order to give context to their own connection to the military and to their countertransference responses.

MEREDITH MCMACKIN, PHD, LMHCA

Meredith earned her undergraduate and master's of fine arts degrees in studio art and taught art in high school and college for many years before entering the field of art therapy. With the death of her son in the war in Iraq, she became drawn to work with veterans and use her background in art towards the goal of bringing peace and healing to others impacted by the trauma of war. Meredith earned her master's in art therapy and doctorate in art education from Florida State University. Inspired by her work with veterans, Meredith focused her dissertation research on papermaking with student veterans in transition. Meredith now lives in Vancouver, Washington, working as an art therapist and mental health counselor.

My personal connection with veterans was what inspired me to become an art therapist. I remember the moment years ago when I had the thought "I really want to work with veterans." And then I thought, "But I don't want to leave all my years of art behind." And then it clicked: "Of course, art therapy!" It was the light bulb moment that changed my life in many wonderful ways. It wouldn't have happened, however, if my older son, my first-born child hadn't given his life in service in Iraq. In fact, before Julian joined the Marines, I had never really felt a connection to the military, although my father was a co-pilot in the Army Air Corps during World War II.

I learned a lot more about the military after Julian joined up. I learned that people join the military for a variety of reasons. For my son, the military was something, that for some reason, he'd been drawn to since childhood. Later, when he struggled with anxiety as a teen-ager, it became his ultimate challenge to prove to himself his own inner strength. And he certainly did. I remember seeing a changed young man at his graduation from boot camp. He was *so* proud of himself; it was clear to see. I knew then that he had made the right decision for himself. When he was killed by an improvised explosive device three years later, my life changed forever. Now, when I think about my life, I frame it by whether it was when Julian was in the world, or after he died.

I floundered for several years after his death, trying to find mean-ingful work I could do in his honor. The thought that kept repeating in my mind was "What can I do to help bring more peace to this planet?" I had seen how many people, including his fellow service members, had suffered, from just his death. I thought of all the thousands who had died in the wars in Iraq and Afghanistan, and I sensed a massive aching wound in the world. I made my own response art, which was personally healing, but I didn't feel it was enough to make a difference in the world. My first involvement with veterans was as an advisor for a student veterans' organization at Florida State University. It was so rewarding, and personally comforting, to me. Being around these young veterans somehow made me feel closer to Julian; it felt familiar. I felt I had some insight into what they had gone through, and knew a little about the military culture from a family perspective. Most all of the student veterans I knew had also lost at least one friend or witnessed death in battle and I felt a connection through our grief and loss.

My experience using art with veterans began while I was in my graduate art therapy program. When veterans knew I was a Gold Star Mother (having lost a son while in active service), I felt a reciprocal connection. I found myself trying to model resiliency and show that there is hope and growth that can happen following traumatic loss. I encountered many veterans expressing survivors' guilt and I hoped through caring for them and appreciating their service, I might relieve some of their guilt.

I don't always share my story with the veterans I work with—only if it feels appropriate or if they ask. But over the years, I have come to feel more comfortable being upfront with my connection to the military and the personal cost of war. It has become easier to talk about; however, I often experience a pounding in my chest and sometimes tear up as I initially talk about my son's death. Once it's out in the open, however, I feel I can be more myself and it explains my purpose and why I chose to be there.

I am aware of my triggers in working with combat veterans in particular, and struggle sometimes with details they share, especially related to bombs and violent death. But I also believe my personal experience has made me more sensitive to veterans' challenges with trauma and grief, even though it can be more emotionally challenging. At the same time, when I'm working with veterans, I feel as if we are going through the process of healing together, which creates a meaningful bond.

As always when working with clients, I believe it is crucial to be aware of countertransference towards clients, and to tease out our emotional reactions during therapy sessions. Although I am aware of my challenges of working with veterans, and the emotional toll it sometimes takes, I have developed a sense of familiarity and comfort in working with this population. I am learning to be mindful of my emotions and triggers while engaging with veterans. When I feel triggered, it can be challenging to stay focused on the client and listen carefully to their feelings, to what they express, watching for visual cues, and perhaps what they avoid sharing. I need to remember that their military experience and their reactions and belief systems may be very different from my own, and I need to be aware of not making assumptions. I continue to practice mindful awareness of my countertransference and make a conscious effort to listen carefully to the veterans' words and emotional state, and respond to their needs, not my own.

GIOIA CHILTON, PHD., ATR-BC, LCPAT, CSAC

Gioia is a registered and board-certified art therapist with over 25 years of experience in using the creative arts in healing. She holds licenses as a clinical professional art therapist (LCPAT) in Maryland and a certified substance abuse counselor (CSAC) in Virginia. Gioia works with active-duty military service members and their families in the Washington, DC area, with the National Endowment for the Arts Creative Forces. Gioia has written numerous academic articles and book chapters and completed award-winning original research on the expression of positive emotions through art. She is co-author of the textbook, Positive Art Therapy Theory and Practice: Integrating Positive Psychology with Art Therapy, *published by Routledge in 2018.*

The opinions and assertions contained herein are the private views of the author and are not to be construed as official or as reflecting the views of the Department of Defense or the U.S. Government. This document was created free of branding or market affiliations. The author is operating solely as a contributor.

As an art therapist who has been working with diverse populations for 25 years, I found this last year intriguing. It was my first year working with a military-connected population as part of a multidiscipline, integrative health clinic on a military base very near my house. Initially, I was awed and a bit humbled by the service members, veterans, and military families who came to art therapy. Although I had worked with many professional adults in the past in addiction treatment, community college, and health-care settings, including with a few veterans here and there, I was almost intimidated by the high level of functioning I saw before me. These service members were either at the end of stellar 20- or 25-year military careers, or were currently on active-duty service. They were clearly smarter than me and more competent in many ways, and many were likely my neighbors. It was only through our in-depth discussions regarding their art that I began to understand how serious mental and physical health concerns resulting from mild traumatic brain injury and post-traumatic stress were impacting their lives in many ways.

My countertransference included my fuzzy fantasies of what military service entails, mostly informed by pop culture. While my father had served in World War II, most of my life I just thought of his profession as an attorney, as his military service seemed long ago and of minor importance. It was only later, at the end of his life, when he stated a preference for a simple VA-provided headstone, with his military rank on it, that I realized his service had been very important to him. I think he would be proud of my work with the military, and this certainly motivates me and infuses my positive transference towards the service members with whom I work.

Starting this job, I searched for where I could find deeper under-standing regarding military culture. I did have an ace up my sleeve that loomed large in my life: 23 years ago, I'd married into a military family. My husband was a "military brat" (and, we often laugh, emphasis on the brat!) who grew up on several Army military bases across the United States. His father—inspired to serve because of the death of *his* father, a fighter pilot in World War II—retired as a full colonel after he served for 30 years. He helped maintain peace in Korea, until his heart attack sent him home to support the Army through military contracting work for another 15 years until his retirement. Today, my father-in-law is an incredibly generous, jovial man who wears flamboyant outfits where the stars-and-stripes are well represented.

I am in a process of learning the difference between what military culture is, and what is unique to my husband's family culture. Some things, though, are clearer to me now, such as the generational impact of war trauma on families and the challenges military families endure. For my husband and his sister, moving over and over again, breaking important relational attachments with friends, colleagues, and teachers, having their father deployed, their mom shouldering important but unrecognized military spouse duties, the weight the shadow of their grandfather's death as a war-hero cast on the family—all were experiences that both adversely impacted their childhood and adulthood, and created strengths that manifest in our family today. As Scandlyn and Hautzinger (2014) note, war's violence does not stay on the battlefield but affects us all—soldiers, military families, children, civilians alike—cascading over decades and generations.

Early in my art therapy career, 20 years ago, I spent several years doing intensive prejudice-reduction diversity training work, where I became more conscious of my identity and privilege as a white straight woman who grew up with plenty of financial resources. Now, I dimly start to understand that, as with white privilege, I also hold "civilian" privilege. This job as an art therapist with the military suddenly gives me a new understanding of an identity I've always had before, but never noticed until now. It is a really important way that I am different from my clients that I never previously thought much about. I have never consciously had to carry much of the weight of war. I now approach my clients knowing they may have transference towards me related to this identify difference. They may wonder, "How can this civilian understand me and my experience?" Meanwhile, I am just beginning to understand my "civilian" identity and my identity as part of a military family.

As I grow in my consciousness of different kinds of privilege, I also understand how the hero myth surrounding soldiers impacts their transference and my countertransference. You know how the hero myth goes: Heroes are heroes. They protect others. They don't get injured, express suffering, or need help. They don't talk about their feelings. They don't make art. In movies, the comic book hero's struggle is always more about beating the bad guys than it is about communicating their pain with loved ones and themselves.

As I see it, whether my clients are male or female (80% are male), they have been socialized into performing a gendered role which constricts their ability to ask for and accept help. Additionally, the messages they received about how to behave—as a man, solider, sailor, ranger, marine, airman—can limit self-expression. Sometimes this silence is due to the fact they literally cannot disclose information because of national security concerns, but at other times this constriction helps compartmentalize trauma. This silent hero myth is part of the larger concept of *militarized masculinity*, how governments require their military to be able to conduct sanctioned violence (and thus enforce power), which ultimately negatively impacts global society (Bulmer & Eichler, 2017). It's important to note that masculinity is violent not by nature, and the reality of maimed and injured service members, veterans, female and gay service members all unmake this stereotypical militarized masculine identity. But on the individual level, back in the art therapy studio, it's just my patient and me in my gendered role as art therapist, trying to communicate across broad swaths of different experiences and understandings regarding how to be a human, not a hero.

Freedom is not free, they say, in an effort to raise awareness of the cost in human suffering paid by our veterans and military. But also in the military, from my perspective as a civilian, there is not a lot of room to be free, have personal choice and autonomy. Those who are fighting for "freedom" don't get to have as much of it as us "civilians" do. So sometimes, as I encourage service members to just let go and create, I'm aware that this is antithetical to the military culture they are living. Art therapy, and the creative arts therapies more broadly, is at its core about human liberation though healing uses of creativity, and is (I hope) empowering freedom. This message conflicts with the ethos of militarized masculinity.

As you can tell from my musings, for me, it kicks up all sorts of confusion as I sort through my positive and negative transference. Part of me admires my clients, many of whom are what we would call genuine "American heroes" (though they might reject that heavy, unhelpful label). Part of me feels sympathy (or—God, I hope not—even pity) for their suffering and their visible and invisible injuries. Part of me feels incomprehension as I try to understand what they've been through, knowing I will never be able to *really* understand. But I've been a therapist for a long time now. I've learned that if I put most of that aside and can listen well and be present, most of the time no matter the differences of our various experiences, identities, and transferences, we can form that deeply intimate human connection where the true art therapy healing happens. And it's a good thing.

I see many service members and family members really taking to art therapy with gusto, using their well-honed self-discipline and problem-solving skills to create thoughtful, powerful, and well-made works of art that are highly expressive of their emotional life. And, as I live close to my in-laws and see the strengths and wonderful characteristics of a creative and vital veteran and his spouse every day, I'm intimately aware of the enduring nature of the strengths and resilience of those who've served. Now, I begin to understand in new ways war's impact on my father, father-in-law, my immediate family and myself. And every day, I grow in understanding my own complicated countertransference towards those whom I serve as an art therapist.

PETER BUOTTE

Peter is a board-certified art therapist working on an active-duty military base. Since December 2016, he has created an environment to support individual and group art therapy sessions for service members who have post-traumatic stress and/or mild traumatic brain injury. His clinical approach is strengths-based and cognitive processing. He completed 27 years of military service in the U.S. Army, culminating as a Lieutenant Colonel with five combat tours overseas. Peter is an active artist who trained at the School of Visual Arts in New York and the Ecole de Beaux Arts in Paris

Each of the three patients mentioned in this paper has voluntarily signed an art image release agreement.

Sigmund Freud first identified countertransference in *The Future Prospects of Psycho-Analytic Therapy* published in 1910. He considered countertransference the patient's influence on the therapist's feelings and a potential barrier to treatment progress. This unconscious phenomenon continues today. The contemporary view of countertransference is as an interpersonal trigger that can be instigated by either the patient or therapist (Gabbard, 1999). Emotional countertransference can range from humor and love, to hate, fear, or anger. As an internal dynamic, countertransference is a useful mental, emotional, and somatic experience which allows insight into, and empathy for, the plight of the other.

During the journey from graduate student, to supervisee, to board-certified art therapist, I have found countertransference an important nuance to learn. Here I will recount three specific instances of my countertransference with active-duty service members. I will focus on three patients, two in separate art therapy groups and one in an individual session.

Client AB

One patient (I will call him AB) is a mid-level officer with four combat tours whose specialty is vehicle recovery and maintenance. To his credit, he had been in two previous post-traumatic stress disorder (PTSD) groups and processed some aspects of his combat trauma. Yet, he was still in his process. As the ranking senior, AB became a focal point and protectively allowed access to other group members only through him. He displayed this trait immediately in the first group session. AB proclaimed to me and to five fellow patients to know "more about PTSD and traumatic brain injury than anyone, including the providers, so you can't trust them." This set up a classic splitting situation of service members versus providers. To assure the group, I disclosed that I too had been a fellow service member with multiple combat tours, and that

I supported their successful treatment. To move the session forward, I invited the service members to draw themselves "in a safe place."

During the second group session, I invited each member to draw a recurring thought. One member of the group was stuck, had tears in her eyes, and could not start her drawing. A natural leader, AB took charge and told her, "That's okay if you can't do it, just think of your safe place that you drew last session." AB then told me that she "was not going to make the artwork." It seemed that AB was playing the role of a gatekeeper and assuming the role of a peer counselor or therapist. AB's comment instigated internal thoughts in me: "Who does AB think he is?" and "Since when is he in charge?" There seemed to be a subtle challenge to the power dynamic. I invited AB "to please continue your work. I will tend to the patient who is having difficulty."

This situation made me recall a past occurrence when I was a graduate student and had been formally counseled to "accept the role as a student, since you are not a therapist." The emotional response was the feeling of not being empowered. As a point of empathy, my comments affected AB so that he did not feel empowered as a patient. For the remainder of the session, AB shut down, made no eye contact, and was quiet. Yet AB did produce a drawing of a recurring thought, below (Figure 8.1).

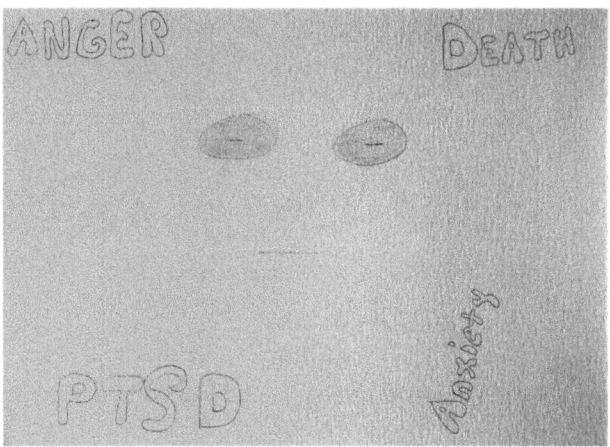

Figure 8.1: AB's drawing

It shows a face with red eyes, closed and crying, and no noticeable boundaries. The words Anger, Death, PTSD and Anxiety are in each corner of the composition. The artwork suggests that AB still had a number of things to be processed. Visually, the lack of boundaries may indicate a lack of protection from, and enmeshment with, these traumatic conditions. It may also suggest a parallel in his lack of boundaries between the role of patient and therapist. The minimal use of color suggests a lack of affect, and the closed mouth suggests difficulty expressing the affect that is there. At the end of the session, I stated again that I supported everyone's successful treatment. After the session, I apologized to AB individually and committed to helping him diminish the recurring thoughts indicated in his drawing. AB accepted my offer.

The same week, I discussed this situation in supervision. To probe the interaction, I made response art with oil pastels and watercolor on paper (Figure 8.2).

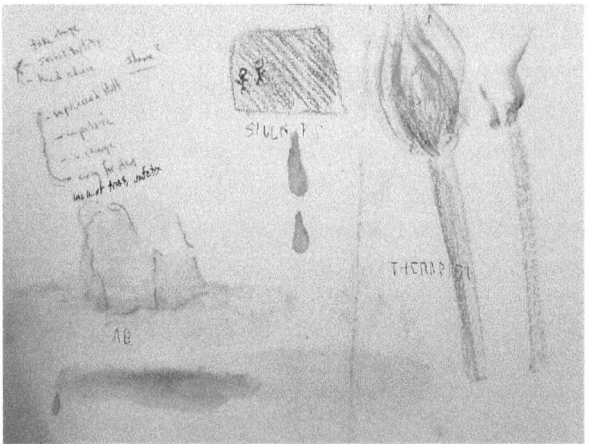

Figure 8.2: My response art

In the middle is a red square with tears, which symbolizes the patient who was stuck. To the right is the therapist symbolized as a flame. My response had a negative effect, AB is represented as an ice cube—cold, distant, and melting. Next to the flame is an extinguished match, symbolizing the apology.

After intensive outpatient program graduation, AB requested to continue art therapy in individual sessions. As a therapeutic goal, AB wanted to process grief and loss by creating a memory box. For the first time in 12 years, AB wanted to honor three fallen battle buddies that he had lost in 2007 in Iraq. Over a period of six sessions, AB gathered and assembled materials, including a wooden cigar box, color felt, identity tags, and printed photos. His memory box can be seen in Figure 8.3.

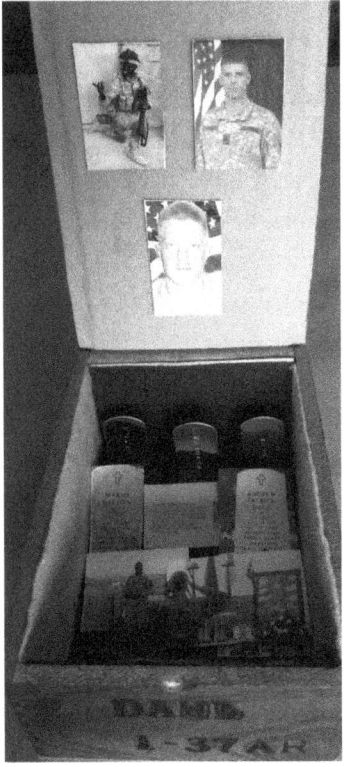

Figure 8.3: AB's memory box

During its creation, AB was able to recount stories of seeing each soldier before going out on their respective fatal missions. Each session he was able to emote and further relieve the emotional baggage that he had carried for too long. With the memory box as a tangible container to hold his losses, AB confided that art therapy sessions became the safe place to disclose what he never could before. In spite of the difficult early sessions, both AB and I were able to gain trust, surmount the initial countertransference, and arrive at what AB deeply desired to process.

Client BC

A small number of patients verbally pushback in session. Here I will highlight one patient, alias BC, who vigorously enabled disruption and repeated countertransferences in me. BC is a mid-grade officer at the end of a 20-year career in charge of a unit of undeployable soldiers, including himself. As a matter of protocol, the very first art invitation offered in session is "Draw yourself in a safe place." As materials were being passed out, BC loudly said, "I don't have a safe space!" All five other patients stopped and looked at him. Since BC was of senior rank-ing, no one made a comment. In this instance, my countertransference was a sense of urgency to decompress the situation and find an activity to soothe BC, who seemed angry and resistant. I said to the group, "If you have a real safe place, that is okay. If you do not, you can imagine one and that is okay, too." Encouraging the other patients to start, I offered BC an alternative activity. Again, BC loudly said, "I don't want any materials and I'm not making anything!" This further elevated the urgency to calm the tension in the patient, his teammates, and myself. I then offered a number of magazines to choose from; BC accepted. This offered a respite for all involved. For 40 minutes, BC remained calm, read magazines, and did not socialize with the other group members. With minutes remaining before the clean-up and close of the session, BC quickly sketched with pencil on paper a small figure, showing no facial affect, isolated in a boat. Oil pastels completed the water and night sky (Figure 8.4).

"There, I did something," BC said. There seemed to be a combination of pushback, passive aggression, and last-minute minimal effort all in one. The artwork suggests isolation and difficulty showing emotion even in a safe space. The suspended figure in the boat suggests a lack of grounding and safety. As non-verbal communication, BC's artwork spoke clearly on behalf of the patient and became a point of empathy for me.

During a third group session, I offered an art invitation to do an emotional inventory by creating a heart chart. This self-assessment uses the concept of a pie chart in the shape of a heart. However, BC said, "I don't have a heart and if I did it would be black." This comment offered some insight into BC's perceived emotional state and self-esteem, as did his heart chart (Figure 8.5).

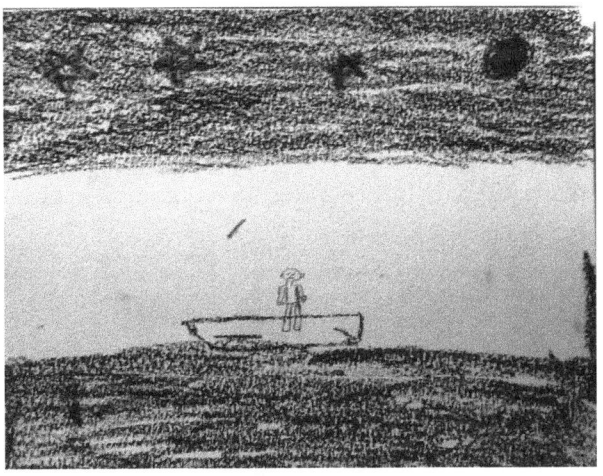

Figure 8.4: BC's drawing

1. Emotional hurt	70%	85%			
2. Eager	95%	90%			
3. Inadequate	65%	70%			
4. Overwhelmed	98%	100%			
5. Depressed	90%	95%			
6. Distant	80%	90%			
7. Anger	100%	95%			
8. Hopeful	40%	40%			

Figure 8.5: BC's heart chart

Instead of a heart to contain his emotions, BC used a ruler and made a grid in black marker. The grid speaks of rigid thinking and the need for containment. The use of one color speaks of difficulty with emotional regulation. BC's baseline assessment indicates anger and feeling overwhelmed as his top two emotions. Beyond 100 percent, the total percentage of emotions adds to 638 percent. Weeks later, on a second review, seven of BC's eight emotions increased in intensity and added up to 655 percent. One emotion, hopeful, continued to trail at a consistent 40 percent.

In the last three weeks of the six-week group, service members make a final art project. They have a choice of collage, mask, memory box, or a hybrid combination of each. BC chose to make a mask in a box, which can be seen in Figure 8.6, below.

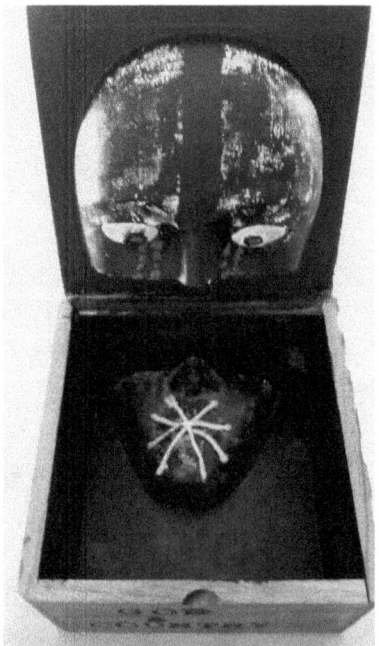

Figure 8.6: BC's mask

The most prevalent colors are black and red, which are indicators of trauma. The mask is split in two, which may suggest a divided self.

The eyes are wide open, reddened, and crying red tears, which metaphorically suggests what BC has seen. The mouth is sealed with an asterisk made of yarn, which may indicate things BC still could not tell.

During individual follow-on sessions, BC admitted that he was depressed because he could no longer deploy, he was angry for not receiving support for his unit, and was anxious about separating and retiring from the service in the near future. While it was non-verbally communicated in his artworks, BC finally was able to put words to his emotions and candidly express them. In his final individual session, he realized that his resistance to making art was actually his resistance to acknowledge and feel his emotions.

Client CD

Another patient, alias CD, is an Infantry non-commissioned officer with 20 years of service and three combat tours. He had been diligently working through loss by making a memory box. However, in his sixth individual session, CD came in visibly angry. He exclaimed that he felt "stressed, stuck, and angry." With flaring nostrils, he said he wanted to "lash out at his First Sergeant." CD's anger caused both an emotional and physical countertransference in me. Internal fear produced an overall tensed bodily response, as if I was anticipating a potential blow. Fear-based internal questions were: "Is he going to hurt me?" "Are all of the sharps (scissors, craft knives) out the patient's reach?" and "Am I the closest to the door in order to escape?" The answers were: I do not know, yes, and yes. The final question was: "What art invitation can I offer to de-escalate the patient's anger and my fear quickly?"

I decided on a bilateral drawing for emotional regulation. Much like push-ups, this drawing requires exertion of the arms, and can last from 5 to 30 minutes depending on the need for emotional release. Physically positioned at the opposite end of the table, I offered CD the opportunity to release the emotions he was feeling in the moment. He asked how. I explained by taping down a 24" x 36" piece of cardboard and using two markers to symbolize two emotions. CD agreed. My heightened response reduced to the level of feeling relieved and willing to proceed.

The cardboard was taped securely to the table and CD selected a red and black marker.

To begin, I led CD in a deep breathing exercise. He then made heavy synchronous and asynchronous gross motor marks for ten minutes and then stopped. Two depleted markers were replaced. After another deep breathing exercise, CD continued to make synchronous and asynchronous gross motor marks for ten more minutes. He then stopped, laid down two depleted markers, and then revealed, "Red was my anger and black was my hatred." CD verbally titled the work "Unexpected" and then said, "I feel much less aggravated." He expressed thanks and appeared to be in a more relaxed, regulated state. In a positive countertransference, I also felt more relaxed and happy for the patient. To close the exercise and to practice coping skills, CD led a final deep breathing exercise.

Final thoughts

Here I have shared three unique instances of countertransference in group and individual settings. With awareness, countertransference is a tool that can deflate an elevated situation, achieve insight into oneself, and gain empathy for the patient. As I continue to identify micro-countertransferences, the better the therapeutic response will be with art materials and creative interventions for patient treatment.

KEVIN D'AUGUSTINE, MA, ATR

Kevin is a prior enlisted service member, having served in the U.S. Marine Corps and U.S. Army, each for five years. Kevin conducts individual and group art therapy sessions at the Naval Medical Center Portsmouth as part of the Creative Forces: National Endowment for the Arts Military Healing Arts Network. He currently supports a substance abuse rehabilitation program, a traumatic brain injury clinic, a crisis stabilization program, and a psychiatric intensive outpatient program.

Please note that I have limited my comments here to those countertransference experiences that relate solely to my military experiences. I do encounter other forms of countertransference, the same as therapists of non-veteran populations, like grief, patient/therapist personality clashes, and conflicting beliefs. Those will not be covered here.

My background

I got into art therapy as a fourth career after a decade in the armed forces, over a decade in the information technology field, and four years as a tattoo artist. The decision to pursue art therapy as a career came about during an existential crisis I experienced in my mid-40s. I was interested in working with service members, veterans, and their families, not only because many of my family members have served or are currently serving, but also because of the support and care my wife and I received following the death of a close family member while he served in the Air Force.

My motivation was to maintain a connection and assist populations that are asked to give so much and are frequently put in harm's way. There are many, many populations deserving of support, and the military was the population with which I wanted to begin my career as a therapist. At the beginning of my art therapy studies, I was aware of the potential for vicarious trauma but I was ignorant as to what transference and countertransference were or how they could play a role in therapeutic relationships. Of course, during my studies and internships, I learned that they are inevitable (Cozolino, 2004). Interesting to me are the triggers I experienced and which I continue to experience in some sessions. To clarify the nature of the transference and countertransference, I must give you a synopsis of my personal history.

Following high school, I served five enlisted years in the Marine Corps. I served in one of the military intelligence fields and manned a lot of desks. It was nothing terribly exciting and definitely not dangerous. I had some good times and bad times. In my first few years of service, I drank a lot of alcohol, which was tolerated, accepted, and sometimes seemingly encouraged by many in the military. Drinking was part of the culture and many young people did it. Sometimes it caused small problems for me, but nothing extreme or lasting. I deployed to

Japan, where I was married, became a father, and divorced within the span of a few years. After my discharge from the Marines and a short attempt at civilian life, I enlisted in the Army out of necessity; other military branches were not accepting prior service enlisted people to join during that period of military cutbacks.

Thus, I served five years in the Army, during which I married for a second time, was discharged from the Army, got custody of my son, received my bachelor's degree in art, and worked in the information technology field. After ten years working in the IT field, in an attempt to do something more art related, I took a four-year hiatus to try my hand at tattooing. I completed a two-year apprenticeship and worked for two years beyond that in a couple of tattoo shops. It was a bizarre world and not satisfying artistically or financially, so I returned to IT work and worked at it, miserably, for two years, and then tragedy struck my family. The sudden loss of a close family member caused me to evaluate my life and what I wanted to do with it before I died. I did not want to live an entire life having done nothing meaningful or satisfying. The sudden loss reminded me that we can rarely predict when we will depart this world and, therefore, if I were going to make a meaningful change in my life, I should do it immediately.

Within a few weeks of the loss, I identified art therapy as a career that would allow me to attempt to get that life of meaning. I spent four years pursuing some missing prerequisites and a graduate art therapy program. During my studies, I interned in a community mental health clinic, a school for adolescents with behavioral and emotional difficulties, and at a military clinic serving military service members with mild traumatic brain injury (TBI) and PTSD. Following graduation, I was hired as a contracted art therapist to support military clinics focused on TBI and PTSD.

Transference/countertransference

Definitions of countertransference vary through psychological texts and, for my examples, I weigh my experiences against the more inclusive definitions. Pearlman and Saakvitne's (1995) liberal interpretation defines countertransference as "any response the therapist has to [his or] her client, positive or negative, conscious or unconscious, spoken or unspoken" (p.22). While stricter definitions limit countertransference to be the therapist's unconscious response to the client (Pearlman & Saakvitne, 1995), I am using the more inclusive definition because I am aware that my conscious reactions (not just my unconscious ones) to my patients do play a significant and regular role within my clinical work.

My case examples are snapshots taken from my work in several military mental health clinics, both as an intern during my art therapy graduate studies and in the work that followed graduation. The clinics include: two TBI/PTSD intensive outpatient programs (IOPs) on military installations in different states, a substance abuse rehabilitation program, a psychiatric intensive outpatient program, and a crisis stabilization outpatient program in a military hospital.

Examples of transference/countertransference
TBI/PTSD CLINICS

I am one of those veterans who does not know how to reply when someone thanks me for my service. I never had to do anything dangerous, I never went to a war zone, and I never even pointed a loaded weapon at a real person. I sat behind a desk for most of my career, analyzed data, and sent intelligence reports to offices and other military units. When I interact with service members now, I weigh the pros and cons of disclosing details of my military service. Sometimes a patient will ask about my service, but more often than not, in the various clinics I support, patients are more concerned with what they are going through than their therapists' histories—understandably. The exception was in the TBI/PTSD clinics that served Special Operations Forces (SOF) members. Special operators include: Navy SEALs, Explosive Ordnance Disposal (EOD) personnel, Marine Raiders, and Army Green Berets. Those folks seemed to move faster in many regards than non-SOF personnel. This trait is likely related to the pace of their work lives in which they have to move and think quickly, looking ahead a few steps at all times, and watch out for ever-present dangers. SOF members have very dangerous jobs and a great many have lost friends and comrades in the line of duty. Also, much of what SOF members do is classified. Because of these reasons, SOF members are all very protective of what they do and of each other.

A side effect of this seems to be that many patients, consciously or not, want to connect with their providers quickly. In the clinical setting, it is no surprise that they will be asked about their injuries—physical, emotional, mental, and spiritual. Answering these questions requires disclosure of some kind, sometimes very sensitive or (for some) embarrassing. Few people are comfortable divulging weaknesses, fears, and shortcomings, and that discomfort is magnified for some SOF members. Many place expectations on themselves to be supermen and superwomen. But most do want to heal, and they understand that relationships with the providers are important in achieving that. So, it is not unusual for patients to question the art therapist (and art therapy intern) about their histories in an effort to assess these providers before sharing sensitive details.

One of the questions I sometimes received was whether I served in the military. Answering this question triggered some countertransference for me. As I said, I was behind a desk for most of my military experience and I was sometimes sensitive about that. The SOF guys often speak of being "blown up" and have scars to show from the shrapnel or the bullets that hit them. Even if they did not have bullet scars, they could all speak of life-threatening situations, not to mention having lost friends. I wanted them to know that I raised my hand and volunteered to serve my country and that I understood a lot of what it is like to be in the military. Though I had not experienced combat, I did have experiences like most military service members involving separation from family, occasional pay problems, changing duty stations often, extreme work hours, working in uncomfortable conditions, living in foreign countries, bad and good commands, training cycles, competing for promotions, and so on.

When I shared the nature of my intelligence job with special operators, I would get a variety of responses. Some would show interest and ask a follow-up question or two and some would acknowledge my response and move on to other topics. Because I was never in harm's way, I sometimes felt a little defensive when the question would arise. Yes, I wanted them to know that I was a brother of sorts, but why? Many questions arose: *What were my insecurities regarding my service? What were my insecurities about being a provider? How could I manage these insecurities while I was becoming an art therapist? What was I looking for in working with this population? How could I use my service to expedite connections with this population?*

After I graduated and worked with this population in a full-time capacity, those questions were slowly answered. With experience came reinforcement that what I was doing was worthwhile and beneficial to others; I was living a life of purpose and meaning. I became less sensitive to the nature of my intelligence work, knowing that the SOF community likely benefited from my efforts from time to time as the intelligence I processed disseminated down to their units. And, I now recognize that not all operators have the "You can't understand unless you've been there" attitude. Though this still happens with the special operators from time to time, I have not had the same feeling of scrutiny from non-SOF client populations. In fact, it is often quite the opposite with other military members, as I have seen in the substance abuse rehabilitation clinic I serve.

SUBSTANCE ABUSE REHABILITATION CLINIC

While holding art therapy sessions in a substance abuse rehabilitation clinic, I sometimes wear an apron to protect my clothing as I am prone to being messy with some materials. But my boring, black apron begged for decoration, so I added some graphic elements to it. The first thing I did was put my name on it, the second was to depict the Marine Corps emblem in red and gold. I removed it within a few weeks as it was a significant source of distraction for patients. I often got questions about my service because a patient would be curious about the emblem. For a little while, it seemed as though it was becoming an opening ritual to art therapy sessions. I did appreciate patients' curiosity, but I did not want the focus to be shifted to me. After a brief period of time, I painted over the Marine Corps emblem and added depictions of things I liked—art tools, wood and metal working tools, and a guitar. My military service still comes up from time to time, but in more of an organic way during personal interactions with individuals and groups, not by placing an emblem on myself for all to see.

Another point of connection between me and many patients is the display of my tattoos. Throughout my military years and afterwards, I got numerous tattoos, many of which run down my arms. I tend to wear my dress shirt sleeves rolled up for comfort or I wear short sleeve shirts when the weather permits. Tattoos are a notable part of military culture and I have never heard any grumbling about mine being visible in military clinical settings. Moon (2015) has suggested that art therapists reflect on their professional appearance, including clothing and tattoos, in terms of appropriateness to the clinical setting and the message these things convey about the art therapist, personally. This should be common sense to professionals, but it is worth repeating. Additionally, my first internship supervisor told me something very useful which helps me decide whether or not to bare my tattoos for others to see. If I choose to expose them, I need to be prepared to talk about them. I certainly believe that image is important to colleagues and patients, so I do exercise common sense and cover up my tattoos for briefings, presentations, and VIP visits. But, during a normal work day, patients and providers galore see my tattoos without blinking an eye. Patients at the substance abuse clinic will ask me about them sometimes, but it is rarely a distraction. In fact, having the tattoos, I believe, has aided in building rapport with individuals and groups because of the prevalence of them in the military culture. Additionally, as a former tattoo artist, my knowledge on the subject has allowed me to speak with patients in an informed way, often providing tips to aid them in thinking through their plans for future tattoos and how to find a skillful artist.

As I stated in my brief history, there was a period of time when I drank alcohol often. It was, like getting tattoos, a part of the military culture. In fact, the Marine Corps' first recruiting site was Tun Tavern in Philadelphia (U.S. Department of Defense, n.d.). While working at the substance abuse clinic, I gave much thought to my history of alcohol consumption. There were certainly periods of time when I would have qualified to be a patient at a program like the one that I now support. The stories I hear from some patients are sometimes similar to ones I lived as a young military service member. I sometimes experience what Moon (2015, p.113) calls the "I've Been There…" form of countertransference when I hear a patient talk about their drinking experiences and the problems that have accompanied them. I sympathize with patients when I hear them say something like "The only reason I'm here is because I got caught." But my sympathy is sometimes accompanied by embarrassment for my past behaviors. Sometimes the stories are so familiar to me that I reflect on those who were affected by my drinking and how foolish, immature, and even clichéd I must have looked to others. Luckily, those days passed, and my consumption waned to reasonable levels. Interestingly, in my year and a half in the clinic, only one patient has asked me if I ever dealt with an addiction. In that moment, I was unsure if I should disclose my experience, but I did offer him a simplified answer. I hoped that in my disclosure he was able to derive some hope that changing behaviors is possible. I had contemplated using some therapy techniques to flush out his real question but went for the authentic, personal approach of simply answering the one he asked. *I-thou, here and now*, as the Gestaltists say.

Another aspect of countertransference that I experience in the clinic is what Moon (2015, p.114) identifies as the "When I Was Your Age…" form of countertransference. I see service members ranging in age from 18 to 50+ with their varying attitudes towards recovery, military service, marriage, responsibility, and just about everything else. I can accept the uniqueness of their attitudes, but it takes work in some cases. Sometimes I take issue with the younger, immature service members who complain about seemingly everything and display a lack of responsibility in many aspects of their lives. Part of me wants to say, "Come on, son! Time to grow up! When I was your age…" followed by whatever I believe I was doing better in my life at their age. Part of this, I know, stems from the disregard I often see for military regulations regarding grooming standards. In the clinic I support, patients wear civilian clothes during their stay, but they are not exempt from military grooming standards. Head and facial hair sometimes go unkempt, often as a form of protest by those who oppose being in treatment. After discussing my feelings with other providers, I have determined that my displeasure comes from the fact that when I was their age, I had to abide by grooming standards despite how I felt, and to see them choosing not to do so is disrespectful to the military service, their fellow service members, and me. I cannot explain why I feel disrespected, I just do. The fact that other prior-service providers feel the same way calms my disdain and I can remind myself that the patient is unique and in need of my support.

One obstacle I have found to handling countertransference is my "stuff"—my troubles and concerns following me to work. When I have trouble leaving my personal distractors at the door, I find it harder to manage countertransference. Another obstacle I find to successful management of countertransference is the attitude of other counselors. In some clinics, there are clinicians who talk down about the difficult patients and who laugh at seemingly outrageous patient difficulties and life choices. It can be easy to fall into those traps and join in with less than professional talk about patients, but I find doing so can skew the way I look at them. This is unnecessary and unfair to a patient. I do my best to keep to the important clinical data and leave the gossip behind.

I think I do a pretty good job of acknowledging when I am experiencing countertransference and how it could affect my counseling. I call it "checking myself." When it does happen, I pursue guidance from other counselors, my art therapy supervisor, and my support network, and I make sure to regularly engage in self-care. It is important for me to continue to ask myself questions that probe my reactions and to continue to look for connections between my thoughts, reactions, and the possible effect on my therapist–patient relationships. Even as I enter my fifth decade of life, I am still learning and am grateful to be able to do so. Entering this new career field has allowed me to learn so many things about myself that I may not have had the occasion to encounter otherwise. About countertransference I have learned that the key is to be honest with oneself and admit where there are opportunities to improve and grow.

References

Abbott, K.A., Shanahan, M.J. & Neufeld, R.W.J. (2013). Artistic tasks outperform non-artistic tasks for stress reduction. *Art Therapy, 30*(2), 71–78.

Allen, P.B. (1995). *Art is a Way of Knowing: A Guide to Self-Knowledge and Spiritual Fulfillment Through Creativity.* Boston, MA: Shambhala Publications.

Allen, P.B. (2005). *Art Is a Spiritual Path: Engaging the Sacred through the Practice of Art and Writing.* Boston, MA: Shambhala Publications.

American Alliance of Museums (2018). *Museums on Call: How Museums are Addressing Health Issues.* Retrieved on 12 May 2020 from www.aam-us.org/wp-content/uploads/2018/01/museums-on-call.pdf.

American Psychiatric Association (2013). *Diagnostic and Statistical Manual of Mental Disorders* (5th ed.) (*DSM-5*). Washington, DC: American Psychiatric Publishing.

American Psychiatric Association (2017). *What is Post-Traumatic Stress Disorder?* Retrieved on 12 May 2020 from www.psychiatry.org/patients-families/ptsd/what-is-ptsd.

American Psychological Association (2014). *The Road to Resilience.* Washington, DC: American Psychological Association. Retrieved on 12 May 2020 from www.apa.org/helpcenter/road-resilience.aspx.

Anderson, F.E. (1995). Catharsis and empowerment group clay work with incest survivors. *The Arts in Psychotherapy, 22*(5) 413–428.

Anderson, G. (Ed.). (2004). *Reinventing the museum: Historical and contemporary perspectives on the paradigm shift.* Landham, MA: Altamira Press.

Avrahami, D. (2008). Visual art therapy's unique contributions in the treatment of post-traumatic stress disorders. *Journal of Trauma & Dissociation, 6*(4), 5–38, doi:10.1300/j229v06n04_02.

Baxter Magolda, M. (2007). Self-authorship: The foundation for twenty-first-century education. *New Directions for Teaching and Learning, 109,* 69–83.

Becker, H. & McCall, M. (1990). *Symbolic Interaction and Cultural Studies.* Chicago, IL: The University of Chicago Press.

Bell, C. & Robbins, S.J. (2007). Effect of art production on negative mood. *Art Therapy: Journal of the American Art Therapy Association, 24*(2), 71–75.

Benight, C. & Bandura, A. (2004). Social cognitive theory of post-traumatic recovery: The role of perceived self-efficacy. *Behaviour Research and Therapy, 42,* 1129–1148.

Berberian, M., Walker, M.S. & Kaimal, G. (2018). "Master My Demons": Art therapy montage paintings by active-duty military service members with traumatic brain injury and post-traumatic stress. *Medical Humanities*, 1–8. doi.org/10.1136/medhum-2018-011493.

Berkowitz, S. (1990). Art therapy with a Vietnam veteran who has post traumatic stress. *Pratt Institute Creative Arts Therapy Review, 11*, 47–62.

Berman, J. (2015). In the end, it seems like we're more human. *Death Studies, 39*(8), 515–517. doi.org/10.1080/07481187.2014.975053.

Betensky, M. G. (1987). Phenomenology of therapeutic art expression and art-therapy. In J. A. Rubin (Ed.), *Approaches to art-therapy: Theory and technique*. New York: Brunner/Mazel.

Betensky, M.G. (2001). Phenomenological Art Therapy. In J. Rubin (ed.), *Approaches to Art Therapy: Theory and Technique* (pp.121–133). New York, NY: Taylor & Francis.

Blumer, H. (1969). The Methodological Position of Symbolic Interactionism. In H. Blumer (ed.), *Symbolic Interactionism: Perspective and Method*. Englewood Cliffs, NJ: Prentice-Hall.

Braitman, A.L., Hamrick, H.C., Ehike, S., Battles, A.R. *et al.* (2018). Psychometric properties of a modified Moral Injury Questionnaire in a military population. *Traumatology, 24*(4), 301–312.

British Association of Art Therapists (BAAT). (2013). Art therapists working with museums and galleries. Retrieved on 12 May 2020 from www.atmag.org/wp-content/uploads/2013/11/AT-and-museums-handout.pdf.

Bryan, C.J., Bryan, A.O., Anestis, M.D., Anestis, J.C. *et al.* (2015). Measuring moral injury: Psychometric properties of the moral injury events scale in two military samples. *Assessment, 23*(5), 557–570.

Bryden, C. (2019). The Narrative Self in the Lived Experience of Dementia. In F. Gibson (ed.), *International Perspectives on Reminiscence, Life Review and Life Story Work*. London: Jessica Kingsley Publishers.

Bulmer, S. & Eichler, M. (2017). Unmaking militarized masculinity: Veterans and the project of military-to-civilian transition. *Critical Military Studies, 3*(2), 161–181.

Butler, T. & Fuhriman, A. (1983). Curative factors in group therapy: A review of the recent literature. *Journal of Small Group Behavior, 14*(2), 131–142. doi:10.1177/104649648301400201.

Callahan, J.L. (2009). Manifestations of power and control: Training as the catalyst for scandal at the United States Air Force Academy. *Violence Against Women, 15*(1), 1149–1168, doi:10.1177/1077801209344341.

Canto, A.I., Mc Mackin, M.L., Hayden, S.C., Jeffreymo, K.A. & Osborn, D.S. (2015). Military veterans: Creative counseling with student veterans. *Journal of Poetry Therapy, 28*(2), 147–163.

Capacchione, L. (1989). *The Creative Journal, The Art of Finding Yourself*. Van Nuys, CA: Newcastle Publishing.

Capacchione, L. (2002). *The Creative Journal: The Art of Finding Yourself* (2nd ed.). Franklin Lakes, NJ: New Page Books.

Cappeliez, P. (2019). Self Reminiscences of Clinically Depressed Older Adults and the Triparte Functional Model Revisited. In F. Gibson (ed.), *International Perspectives on Reminiscence, Life Review and Life Story Work*. London: Jessica Kingsley Publishers.

Catherall, D.R. & Lane, C. (1990). Warrior therapist: Vets treating vets. *Journal of Traumatic Stress, 5*(1), 19–36.

Center for Substance Abuse Treatment, (2014). Exhibit 1.3–4, DSM-5 Diagnostic Criteria for PTSD. *Trauma-Informed Care in Behavioral Health Services*. Rockville (MD): Substance Abuse and Mental Health Services Administration. (Treatment Improvement Protocol (TIP) Series, No. 57.) Retrieved on 12 May 2020 from www.ncbi.nlm.nih.gov/books/NBK207191/box/part1_ch3.box16.

Chatterjee, H. & Noble, G. (2016). *Museums, Health and Well-Being*. New York, NY: Routledge.

Cloitre, M., Jackson, C. & Schmidt, J.A. (2016). Case reports: STAIR for strengthening social support and relationships among veterans with military sexual trauma. *Military Medicine, 181*, e183–e187.

Cloitre, M. & Schmidt, J.A. (2015). STAIR Narrative Therapy. In U. Schnuder & M. Cloitre (eds), *Evidence Based Treatments for Trauma-Related Psychological Disorders: A Practical Guide for Clinicians*. doi: 10.1007/978-3-319-07109-1_14.

Coll, J.E. & Weiss, E.L. (2013). Transitioning Veterans into Civilian Life. In A. Rubin, E. Weiss & J.E. Coll (eds), *Handbook of Military Social Work*. Hoboken, NJ: Wiley.

Collie, K., Backos, A., Malchiodi, C. & Spiegel, D. (2006). Art therapy for combat-related PTSD: Recommendations for research and practice. *Art Therapy, 23*(4), 157–164. doi:10.1080/07421656.2006.10129335.

Cozolino, L.J. (2004). *The Making of a Therapist: A Practical Guide for the Inner Journey*. New York, NY: W.W. Norton.

Csamanski-Cohen, J. & Weihs, K.L. (2016). The bodymind model: A platform for studying the mechanisms of change induced by art therapy. *The Arts in Psychotherapy, 51*, 63–71.

Csikszentmihalyi, M. (2017). *Why We Enjoy Making Art*. American Art Therapy Conference Presentation. Albuquerque, NM.

Curl, K. (2008). Assessing stress reduction as a function of artistic creation and cognitive focus. *Art Therapy: Journal of the American Art Therapy Association, 25*(4), 164–169. doi:10.1080/07421656.2008.10129550.

Currier, J.M., Farnsworth, J.K., Drescher, K.D., McDermott, R.C., Sims, B.M. & Albright, D.L. (2017a). Development and evaluation of the Expressions of Moral Injury Scale—Military Version. *Clinical Psychology & Psychotherapy, 25*, 474–488.

Currier, J.M., Holland, J.M., Drescher, K. & Foy, D. (2015). Initial psychometric evaluation of the moral injury questionnaire – military version. *Clinical Psychology and Psychotherapy, 22*, 54–63. (Published online 10 September 2013, Copyright 2013 John Wiley & Sons).

Currier, J.M., Stefurak, T., Carroll, T.D. & Shatto, E.H. (2017b). Applying Trauma-Informed Care to community-based mental health services for military veterans. *Best Practices in Mental Health, 13*(1), 47–64.

Dardis, C.M., Reinhardt, K.M., Foynes, M.M., Medoff, N.E. & Street, A.E. (2018). Who are you going to tell? Who's going to believe you?: Women's experiences disclosing military sexual trauma. *Psychology of Women Quarterly, 42*(4), 414–429. doi.org/10.1177/0361684318796783.

David, W.S., Simpson, T.L. & Cotton, A.J. (2006). Taking charge: A pilot curriculum of self-defense and personal safety training for female veterans with PTSD because of military sexual trauma. *Journal of Interpersonal Violence, 21*(4), 555–565, doi:10.1177/0886260505285723.

Davison, E.H., Kaiser, A.P., Spiro, A., Moye, J., King, L.A. & King, D.W. (2016). From late-onset stress symptomatology to later-adulthood trauma reengagement in aging combat veterans: Taking a broader view. *Gerontologist, 56*(1), 14–21. doi.org/10.1093/geront/gnv097.

DeLucia, J.M., (2016). Art therapy services to support veterans' transition to civilian life: The studio and the gallery. *Art Therapy, 33*(1), 4–12.

DiRamio, D. & Jarvis, K. (2011). Veterans in higher education: When Johnny and Jane come marching to campus. *ASHE Higher Education Report, 37*(3) 1–114.

Dohrenwend, B.P., Turner, J.B., Turse, N.A., Adams, B.G., Koenen, K.C. & Marshall R. (2006). The psychological risks of Vietnam for US veterans: A revisit with new data and methods. *Science, 313*(5789): 979–982.

Drake, J.E., Coleman, K. & Winner, E. (2011). Short-term mood repair through art: Effects of medium and strategy. *Art Therapy, 28*(1), 26–30.

Drescher, K.D., Foy, D.W., Kelly, C., Leshner, A., Schutz, K. & Litz, B. (2011). An exploration of the viability and usefulness of the construct of moral injury in war veterans. *Traumatology, 17*(1), 8–13.

Dursun, S. & Watkins, K. (2018). Moral injury: What we know and what we need to know. *Military Behavioral Health, 6*(2), 121–126. doi:10.1080/21635781.2018.1454365.

Duttweiler, R. (2020). Here's what you need to know about reintegration. Retrieved on 12 May 2020 from www.military.com/spouse/military-deployment/reintegration/returning-to-home-life-after-deployment.html.

Eibner, C. (2008). *Fight now, pay later: The future costs of funding the Iraq war.* Hearing before the Joint Economic Committee, 110th Congress (2008) (Testimony of Christine Eibner). Retrieved on 12 May 2020 from www.rand.org/content/dam/rand/pubs/testimonies/2008/RAND_CT309.pdf.

Elkis-Abuhoff, D.L. & Gaydos, M. (2018). Medical art therapy research moves forward: A review of clay manipulation with Parkinson's disease. *Art Therapy, 35*(2), 68–76. doi.org/10.1080/07421656.2018.1483162.

Farnsworth, J.K., Drescher, K.D., Evans, W. & Walser, R.D. (2017). A functional approach to understanding and treating military-related moral injury. *Journal of Contextual Behavioral Science, 6*, 391–397.

Fincher, S. (1989). *Creating Mandalas.* Boston, MA: Shambhala Publishers.

Fish, B.J. (2019). Response art in art therapy: Historical and contemporary overview. *Art Therapy: Journal of the American Art Therapy Association, 36*(3), 122–132.

Fivush, R. & Booker, J.A. (2019). Developmental Foundations of Lifelong Reminiscing. In F. Gibson (ed.), *International Perspectives on Reminiscence, Life Review and Life Story Work.* London: Jessica Kingsley Publishers.

Florida State University. 2019. *Museum Education and Visitor-Centered Curation (EC)*. Retrieved on 12 May 2020 from https://arted.fsu.edu/programs/ec.

Foley, D.D. (n.d.). *Courage Group: Treating Sexual Trauma Among Veterans in Outpatient Group Psychotherapy*. Retrieved on 12 May 2020 from www.mirecc.va.gov/visn16/courage-group-manual.asp.

Frankel, V. (1959, 2006). *Man's Search for Meaning*. Boston, MA: Beacon Press.

Furman, L.R. (2013). *Ethics in Art Therapy: Challenging Topics for a Complex Modality*. London: Jessica Kingsley Publishers.

Freud, S. (1910). The future prospects of psycho-analytic therapy. In *Collected papers, 2*. London: Hogarth, 1946.

Gabbard, G.O. (1999). *Countertransference Issues in Psychiatric Treatment*. Washington, DC: American Psychiatric Press.

Galloucis, M. & Kaufman, M.E. (1988). Group therapy with Vietnam veterans: A brief review. *Group, 12*(2), 85–102.

Gantt, L.M. & Tinnin, L.W. (2009). Support for a neurobiological view of trauma with implications for art therapy. *The Arts in Psychotherapy, 36*(3), 148–153. doi:10.1016/j.aip.2008.12.005.

Gosselin, P.A. & Gagné, J.P. (2011). Older adults expend more listening effort than young adults recognizing speech in noise. *Journal of Speech, Language, and Hearing Research, 54*(3), 944–958. doi.org/10.1044/1092-4388(2010/10-0069.

Gray, M.J., Schorr, Y., Nash, W., Lebowitz, L. *et al.* (2012). Adaptive Disclosure: An open trial of a novel exposure-based intervention for service members with combat-related psychological stress injuries. *Behavior Therapy, 42*, 407–415.

Hamil, S. (2016). *The Art Museum as a Therapeutic Space*. [Doctoral dissertation.]

Hass-Cohen, N. & Findlay, J.C. (2013). *Art Therapy & The Neurosciences of Relationships, Creativity & Resiliency*. New York, NY: W.W. Norton.

Held, P., Klassen, B.J., Brennan, M.B. & Zalta, A.K. (2017). Using Prolonged Exposure and Cognitive Processing Therapy to treat veterans with moral-injury based PTSD: Two case examples. *Cognitive and Behavioral Practice, 25*(3), 377–390.

Hinz, L.D. (2009). *Expressive Therapies Continuum: A Framework for Using Art in Therapy*. New York, NY: Routledge.

Hoge, C.W. (2010). *Once a Warrior Always a Warrior: Navigating the Transition from Combat to Home—Including Combat Stress, PTSD, and mTBI*. Guilford, CT: Globe Pequot Press.

Holliday, R., Williams, R., Mullen, K., Bird, J. & Suris, A. (2015). The role of cognitive processing therapy in improving functioning, and quality of life in veterans with military sexual trauma-related posttraumatic stress disorder. *Psychological Services, 12*(4), 428–434.

Hunter, D. (1978). *Papermaking: The History and Technique of an Ancient Craft*. New York, NY: Dover Publications.

Husserl, E. (1952). *Ideas*. Norwich: Jarrold and Sons.

Iraq Afghanistan Veterans Association. (n.d.). 2019 Member Survey. Retrieved on 12 May 2020 from https://iava.org/survey2019/IAVA-2019-Member-Survey.pdf.

Johnson, D.R. (2000). Creative Therapies. In E. Foa, T. Keane, M. Friedman & A. Cohen (eds), *Effective Treatments for PTSD: Practice Guidelines from the International Society for Traumatic Stress Studies*. New York, NY: Guilford Press.

Johnson, D.R., Rosenheck, R. & Fontana, A. (1997). Assessing the structure, content, and perceived social climate of residential posttraumatic stress disorder treatment programs. *Journal of Traumatic Stress, 10*(3), 361–376.

Jones, J.P., Walker, M.S., Masino Drass, J. & Kaimal, G. (2018). Art therapy interventions for active duty military service members with post-traumatic stress disorder and traumatic brain injury. *International Journal of Art Therapy, 23*(2), 70-85. doi:10.1080/17454832.2017.1388263.

Kaimal, G., Jones, J.P., Dieterich-Hartwell, R., Acharya, B. & Wang, X. (2019). Evaluation of long- and short-term art therapy interventions in an integrative care setting for military service members with post-traumatic stress and traumatic brain injury. *The Arts in Psychotherapy, 62*, 28–36. doi:10.1016/j.aip.2018.10.003.

Kaimal, G., Ray, K. & Muniz, J. (2016). Reduction of cortisol levels and participants' responses following art making. *Art Therapy, 33*(2), 74–80. doi: 10.1080/07421656.2016.1166832.

Kaimal, G., Walker, M.S., Herres, J., French, L.M. & DeGraba, T.J. (2018). Observational study of associations between visual imagery and measures of depression, anxiety and post-traumatic stress among active-duty military service members with traumatic brain injury at the Walter Reed National Military Medical Center. *BMJ Open, 8*(6), 1–9. doi.org/10.1136/bmjopen-2017-021448.

Kashdan, T.B., Elhai, J.D. & Frueh, B.C. (2006). Anhedonia and emotional numbing in combat veterans with PTSD. *Behavior Research and Therapy, 44*(3), 457–467.

Katz, L.S. (2016). Efficacy of warrior renew group therapy for female veterans who have experienced military sexual trauma. *Psychological Services, 13*(4), 364–372.

Katz, L.S., Cojucar, G., Douglas, S. & Huffman, C. (2014). Renew: An integrative psychotherapy program for women veterans with sexual trauma. *Journal of Contemporary Psychotherapy, 44*, 163–171.

Katz, L.S., Cojucar, G., Hoff, R., Lindl, C., Huffamn, C. & Drew, T. (2015). Longitudinal outcomes of women veterans enrolled in the Renew sexual trauma treatment program. *Journal of Contemporary Psychotherapy, 45*, 143–150.

Katz, L.S., Park, S.E., Cojucar, G., Huffman, C. & Douglas, S. (2016). Improved attachment style for female veterans who graduated Warrior Renew sexual trauma treatment. *Violence and Victims, 31*(4), 680–691.

Kellogg, J. (1984). *Mandala: The Path of Beauty*. Williamsburg, VA: Graphic Publishers of Williamsburg.

Kelly, V. A. 2016. Addiction in the family: What every counsellor needs to know. American Counseling Association. https://doi.org/10.1002/9781119255833.ch5

Kielo, J.B. (1991). Art therapists' countertransference and post-session therapy imagery. *Art Therapy: Journal of the American Art Therapy Association, 8*(2), 14–19.

Kimerling, R., Gima, K., Smith, M.W., Street, A. & Frayne, S. (2007). The Veterans Health Administration and military sexual trauma. *American Journal of Public Health, 97*(12), 2160-2166.

Klein, D.L., (2015). *The Art of War: Examining Museums' Art Therapy Programs for Military Veterans*. [Doctoral dissertation, University of Washington.] Research Works Archive. Retrieved on 12 May 2020 from https://digital.lib.washington.edu/researchworks/handle/1773/33420.

Koenig, H.G., Ames, D., Youssef, N.A., Oliver, J.P. *et al.* (2018a). The Moral Injury Symptom Scale— Military Version. *Journal of Religious Health, 57,* 249–265.

Koenig, H.G., Ames, D., Youssef, N.A., Oliver, J.P. *et al.* (2018b). Screening for moral injury: The Moral Injury Symptoms Scale—Military Version Short Form. *Military Medicine, 183,* e659–e665.

Koenig, H.G., Youssef, N.A. & Pearce, M. (2019). Assessment of moral injury in veterans and active duty military personnel with PTSD: A review. *Frontiers in Psychiatry, 10,* 1–15.

Kopytin, A. & Lebedev, A. (2013). Humor, self-attitude, emotions, and cognitions in group art therapy with war veterans. *Art Therapy, 30*(1), 20–29.

Kulesza, M., Pedersen, E. & Marshall, G. (2015). Help-seeking stigma and mental health treatment seeking among young adult veterans. *Military Behavioral Health, 3*(4), 230–239.

Lancaster, A.R. (1999). Department of Defense sexual harassment research: Historical perspectives and new initiatives. *Military Psychology, 11*(3), 219–231.

Laurel Ridge Treatment Center (2020). *Military Program: Mission Resiliency.* https://laurelridgetc.com/programs/military-dependents/#:~:text=In%20response%20to%20the%20present,dedicated%20to%20treating%20active%20duty.

Levine, P. (1997). *Waking the Tiger Healing Trauma: The Innate Capacity to Transform Overwhelming Experiences.* Berkeley, CA: North Atlantic Books.

Levy, C.E., Spooner, H., Lee, J.B., Sonke, J., Myers, K. & Snow, E., (2018). Telehealth-based creative arts therapy: Transforming mental health and rehabilitation care for rural veterans. *The Arts in Psychotherapy, 57,* 20–26.

Lewis, J.A., Dana, R.Q. & Blevins, G.A. (2015). *Substance Abuse Counseling* (5th ed.). Stamford, CT: Cengage Learning.

Linehan, M.M. (2015). *DBT Skills Training: Handouts and Worksheets* (2nd ed.). New York, NY: Guilford Press.

Litz, B.T., Stein, N., Delaney, E., Lebowitz, L. *et al.* (2009). Moral injury and moral repair in war veterans: A preliminary model and intervention strategy. *Clinical Psychology Review, 29,* 695–706.

Lobban, J. (2014). The invisible wound: Veterans' art therapy. *International Journal of Art Therapy: Formerly Inscape, 19*(1), 3–18.

Lobban, J. (2016). Factors that influence engagement in an inpatient art therapy group for veterans with post-traumatic stress disorder. *International Journal of Art Therapy, 21*(1), 15–22. doi.org/10.1080/17454832.2015.1124899.

Lobban, J. (2017). *Art Therapy with Military Veterans: Trauma and Image.* New York, NY: Taylor & Francis.

Lobban, J. & Murphy, D. (2018). Using art therapy to overcome avoidance in veterans with chronic post-traumatic stress disorder. *International Journal of Art Therapy, 23*(3), 99–114. doi:10.1080/17454832.2017.1397036.

Lobban, J. & Murphy, D. (2019). Understanding the role art therapy can take in treating veterans with chronic post-traumatic stress disorder. *The Arts in Psychotherapy, 62,* 37–44.

Lusebrink, V.B. (2004). Art therapy and the brain: An attempt to understand the underlying processes of art expression in therapy. *Art Therapy: Journal of the American Art Therapy Association, 21*(3), 125–135. doi: 10.1080/07421656.2004.10129496.

Malchiodi, C.A. (2012). Art Therapy with Combat Veterans and Military Personnel. In C. Malchiodi (ed.), *Handbook of Art Therapy* (2nd ed.). New York, NY: Guilford Press.

Mandic-Gajic, G. & Spiric, Z. (2016). Posttraumatic stress disorder and group art therapy: Self expression of traumatic inner world of war veterans. *Vojnosanitetski pregled, 73*(8), 757–763.

Marshall, J. (2011). *Archetypes of Chaos: The Psychological Significance of Chaos and Disorder*. Retrieved on 12 May 2020 from www.academia.edu/1682445/ Archetypes_of_Chaos_The_ Psychological_Significance_of_Chaos_and_Disorder.

McElveen, R. (2007). Using art as therapy. *Vanguard, September–October 2007*, 18–21.

McGonigal, C. (2016). *Powerful Photos Depict Veterans Who Use Art Therapy to Heal*. Retrieved on 12 May 2020 from www.huffpost.com/entry/veterans-art-therapy_n_6526040.

McMackin, M. (2016). *Assessing the Value of Creative Arts Workshops and Hand Papermaking for Student Veterans in Transition*. [Doctoral dissertation, The Florida State University.] DigiNole: FSU's Digital Repository. Retrieved on 12 May 2020 from http://fsu.digital.flvc.org/islandora/object/fsu%3A366094.

Melter, R.H. (2012). Countertransference Experiences of Psychotherapists Conducting Group Psychotherapy with Combat Veterans. [Unpublished doctoral dissertation.] Wright Institute Gradaute School of Psychology.

Melton, A. (2013). Comfort and connectivity: The museum as a healer. *Museums & Social Issues, 8*(1–2), 6–21. doi:10.1179/1559689313Z.0000000003.

Museum of Art. *Museums & Social Issues, 5*(2), 235–249. doi:10.1179/msi.2010.5.2.235.

Merendino, J. & Clark, M. (2010) Accessible wellness workshops at the Philadelphia Merleau-Ponty, M. (2012). *Phenomenology of Perception*. New York, NY: Routledge.

Metropolitan Museum of Art. (2019). *For Visitors with Dementia and their Care Partners*. Retrieved on 12 May 2020 from www.metmuseum.org/events/programs/ access/visitors-with-dementia-and-their-care-partners.

Middleton, K. & Craig, D. (2012). A systematic literature review of PTSD among female veterans from 1990 to 2010. *Social Work in Mental Health, 10*, 233–252, doi:10.1 080/15332985.2011.639929.

Mims, R. (2015). Military veteran use of visual journaling during recovery. *Journal of Poetry Therapy, 28*(2), 1–13, doi:10.1080/08893675.2015.1008737.

Mims, R. & Jones, J. (2019). Disenfranchised Grief: The Impact of Grief in the Military. In M.J.M. Wood, B. Jacobson & H. Cridford (eds), *The International Handbook of Art Therapy in Palliative and Bereavement Care*. New York, NY: Routledge.

Molina, D. (2014). American Council on Education. Center for Policy Research and Strategy. Center for Education Attainment & Innovation. *2011–2012 National Postsecondary Student Aid Study*. Retrieved on 12 May 2020 from www.acenet.edu/ news-room/Documents/Higher-ed-spotlight-undergraduate-student-veterans.pdf.

Monteith, L.L., Bahraini, N.H., Matarazzo, B.B., Soberay, K.A. & Parnitze Smith, C. (2016). Perceptions of institutional betrayal predict suicidal self-directed violence among veterans exposed to military sexual trauma. *Journal of Clinical Psychology, 72*(7), 743–755, doi:10.1002/jclp.22292.

Moon, B.L. (2015). *Ethical Issues in Art Therapy*. (3rd ed.). Springfield, IL: Charles C. Thomas.

Moon, C.H. (2002). *Studio Art Therapy: Cultivating the Artist Identity in the Art Therapist*. London: Jessica Kingsley Publishers.

Morin, R. (2011). *Pew Research Center: Social and Demographic Trends. The Difficult Transition from Military to Civilian Life*. Retrieved on 12 May 2020 from www.pewsocialtrends. org/2011/12/08/the-difficult-transition-from-military-to-civilian-life.

Museum of Modern Art. (n.d.). Meet Me. Retrieved on 12 May 2020 from www.moma. org/visit/accessibility/meetme.

Najavits, L. (2002). *Seeking Safety: A Manual Guide for Treating PTSD and Substance Abuse*. New York, NY: Guilford Press.

Nan, J.K.M. (2016). *Mind-Body Treatment for Depression: Clay Art Therapy with Expressive Therapies Continuum*. American Art Therapy Conference Presentation. Baltimore, MD.

Nash, W.P., Carper, T.L.M., Mills, M.A., Au, T., Goldsmith, A. & Litz, B.T. (2013). Psychometric evaluation of the moral injury events scale. *Military Medicine, 178*(6), 646–652.

National Advisory Council on Vocational Education (1972). Special report on the employment problems of the Vietnam veteran. Washington, DC. Retrieved on 12 May 2020 from https://eric.ed.gov/?id=ED060204.

National Endowment for the Arts (n.d.). *Creative Forces: NEA Military Healing Arts Network*. Retrieved on 12 May 2020 from www.arts.gov/national-initiatives/ creative-forces.

National Initiative for Arts and Health in the Military (2013). *Arts, Health and Wellbeing across the Military Continuum*. Retrieved on 12 May 2020 from www. americansforthearts.org/sites/default/files/pdf/2013/by_program/legislation_and_ policy/art_and_military/ArtsHealthwellbeingWhitePaper.pdf.

National Institute of Mental Health (n.d.) *Post-Traumatic Stress Disorder*. Retrieved on 12 May 2020 from www.nimh.nih.gov/health/publications/post-traumatic-stress-disorder-ptsd/20-mh-8124-ptsd_38054.pdf.

Naudziunas, J. (2013, June). *How to make museums more inviting for kids with autism*. Retrieved on 12 May 2020 from www.npr.org/sections/health-shots/2013/06/18/193092510/how-to-make-museums-more-inviting-for-kids-with-autism.

Nicholls, O. (2020). *Artist spotlight: Adrian Hill, War Artist and Pioneer of Art Therapy*. Sulis Fine Art. Retrieved on 12 May 2020 from www.sulisfineart.com/blog/post/artist-spotlight-adrian-hill-war-artist-pioneer-art-therapy.

Northcut, T.B. & Keinow, A. (2014). The trauma trifecta of military sexual trauma: A case study illustrating the integration of mind and body in clinical work with survivors of MST. *Clinical Social Work Journal, 42*, 247–259, doi: 10.1007/ s10615-014-0479-0.

Ottemiller, D.D. & Awais, Y.J. (2016). A model for art therapists in community-based practice. *Art Therapy: Journal of the American Art Therapy Association, 33*(3), 144–150. doi:10.1080/07421656.2016.1199245

Packard, S. (1980). The history of art therapy education. *Art Education, 33*(4), 10–13.

Palmer, E., Hill, K., Lobban, J. & Murphy, D. (2017). Veterans' perspectives on the acceptability of art therapy: A mixed-methods study. *International Journal of Art Therapy, 22*(3), 132–137.

Parashak, S.T. (2013). The richness that surrounds us: Collaboration of classroom and community for art therapy and art education. *Art Therapy: Journal of the American Art Therapy Association, 14*(4), 241–245.

Partridge, E.E. (2019a). *Art Therapy with Older Adults: Connected and Empowered.* London: Jessica Kingsley Publishers.

Partridge, E.E. (2019b). Dismantling the Gender Binary in Elder Care: Creativity Instead of Craft. In S. Hogan (ed.), *Gender and Difference in the Arts Therapies: Inscribed on the Body.* Abingdon: Routledge.

Patmali, L. (2017). *Art Therapy in Museums.* Retrieved on 12 May 2020 from www.museeum.com/art-therapy-in-museums.

Peacock, K. (2012). Museum education and art therapy: Exploring an innovative partnership. *Art Therapy: Journal of the American Art Therapy Association, 29*(3), 133–137.

Pearlman, L.A. & Saakvitne, K.W. (1995). *Trauma and the Therapist: Countertransference and Vicarious Traumatization in Psychotherapy with Incest Survivors.* New York, NY: W.W. Norton.

Pike, A.A. (2013). The effect of art therapy on cognitive performance among ethnically diverse older adults. *Art Therapy, 30*(4), 159–168. doi.org/10.1080/07421656.201 4.847049.

Porges, S.W. (2019). *Clinical Applications of the Polyvagal Theory.* CMI/Premier Education Solutions.

Protect Our Defenders (2019). *Industry Study Report.* Retrieved on 12 May 2020 from www.protectourdefenders.com/wp-content/uploads/2019/07/Protect_Our_Defenders_Industry_Study.pdf.

Purcell, N., Burkman, K., Keyser, J., Fucella, P. & Maguen, S. (2018a). Healing from moral injury: A qualitative evaluation of the Impact of Killing treatment for combat veterans. *Journal of Aggression, Maltreatment & Trauma, 27*(6), 645–673.

Purcell, N., Griffin, B.J., Burkman, K. & Maguen, S. (2018b). "Opening a door to a new life": The role of forgiveness in healing from moral injury. *Frontiers in Psychiatry, 9,* 498. doi:10.3389/fpsyt.2018.00498.

Purcell, N., Koenig, C.J., Bosch, J. & Maguen, S. (2016). Veterans' perspectives on the psychosocial impact of killing in war. *The Counseling Psychologist, 44*(7), 1062–1099.

Ramirez, J. (2016). A review of art therapy among military service members and veterans with post traumatic stress disorder. *Journal of Military and Veterans' Health, 24*(2).

Rausch, S.L, van der Kolk, B.A., Fisler, R.E. & Alpert, N.M. (1996). A symptom provocation study of posttraumatic stress disorder using positron emission tomography and script-driven imagery. *Archives of General Psychiatry, 53*(5), 380–387. doi:10.001/archpsych.1996.01830050014003.

Ready, D.J., Sylvers, P., Worley, V., Butt, J., Mascaro, N. & Bradley, B. (2012). The impact of group-based exposure therapy on the PTSD and depression of 30 combat veterans. *Psychological Trauma: Theory, Research, Practice and Policy, 4*(1), 84–93, doi:10.1037/a0021997.

Reda, M. (2009). *Between Speaking and Silence: A Study of Quiet Students.* New York, NY: State University of New York Press.

Reger, M., Smolensky, D. & Skopp, N. (2015). Risk of suicide among military service members following Operation Enduring Freedom or Operation Iraqi Freedom deployment and separation from the US military. *JAMA Psychiatry, 72*(6), 561–569. doi:10.1001/jamapsychiatry.2014.3195.

Regev, D., Kurt, H. & Snir, S. (2016). Silence during art therapy: The art therapist's perspective. *International Journal of Art Therapy: Inscape, 21*(3), 86–94. doi.org/10.1080/17454832.2016.1219754.

Resick, P.A., Monson, C.M. & Chard, K.M. (2017). *Cognitive Processing Therapy for PTSD: A Comprehensive Manual.* New York, NY: Guilford Press.

Rogers, N. (2001). Person-Centered Expressive Arts Therapy. In J. Rubin (ed.) *Approaches to Art Therapy: Theory and Technique.* Philadelphia, PA: Bruner/ Routledge.

Rosenblatt, B. (2014). Museum education and art therapy: Promoting wellness in older adults. *Journal of Museum Education, 39*(3), 293–301.

Rozynko, V. & Dondershine, H.E. (1991). Trauma focus group therapy for Vietnam veterans with PTSD. *Psychotherapy, 28*(1), 157–161.

Rubin, J. (1987). *Approaches to Art Therapy Theory and Technique.* New York, NY: Brunner/Mazel Publishers.

Rubin, J.A. (2001). Discovery, Insight, and Art Therapy. In J. Rubin (ed.) *Approaches to Art Therapy: Theory and Technique.* Philadelphia, PA: Bruner/Routledge.

Ruehrwein, B. (2013). The art museum as trauma clinic: A veteran's story. *Conservation & Museum Studies, 8*(1–2), 36–46.

Salom, A. (2011). Reinventing the setting: Art therapy in museums. *Arts in Psychotherapy, 39*(2), 81–85.

Sandmire, D., Gorham, S., Rankin, N. & Grimm (2012). The influence of art making on anxiety: A pilot study. *Art Therapy, 29*(2), 68–73. doi:10.1080/07421656.2012 .683748.

Scandlyn, J. & Hautzinger, S. (2014). *Collective reckoning with the post 9/11 wars on a Colorado homefront.* Paper written as part of Costs of War project. Watson Institute of International Studies: Brown University. Retrieved on 12 May 2020 from https://watson.brown.edu/costsofwar/files/cow/imce/papers/2014/ ScandlynHautzinger%2061615.pdf.

Schaff, P. (2018). Collaborative commemoration: Narratives as transactional memorials to heal the wounds of war and trauma. *Military Behavioural Health, 6*(2), 127–133.

Schlossberg, N. (2011). The challenge of change: The transition model and its applications. *Journal of Employment Counseling, 48*(4), 159–162.

Schnurr, P.P., Lunney, C.A., Bovin, M.J. & Marx, B.P. (2009). Posttraumatic stress disorder and quality of life: Extension of findings to veterans of the wars in Iraq and Afghanistan. *Clinical Psychological Review, 29*, 727–735, doi:10.1016/j. cpr.2009.08.006.

Schorr, Y., Stein, N.R., Maguen, S., Barnes, J.B., Bosch, J. & Litz, B.T. (2018). Sources of moral injury among war veterans: A qualitative evaluation. *Journal of Clinical Psychology, 74*, 2203–2218. doi:10.1002/jclp.22660.

Schwalbe, M. (1996). *Unlocking the Iron Cage: The Men's Movement, Gender Politics, and American Culture.* Oxford: Oxford University Press.

Serlin, D. (2006). The Other Arms Race. In L.J. Davis (ed.), *The Disability Studies Reader* (2nd ed.). New York, NY: Routledge.

Shay, J. (2012). Moral injury. *Intertexts, 16*(2), 57–66. doi:10.1353/itx.2012.0000.

Silverman, L. (2010). *The Social Work of Museums.* New York, NY: Routledge.

Singer, M. (2004). Shame, guilt, self-hatred and remorse in the psychotherapy of Vietnam combat veterans who committed atrocities. *American Journal of Psychotherapy, 58*(4), 377–385.

Sloan, L. (2013). *Your Brain on Art: Art Therapy in a Museum Setting and its Potential at the Rubin Museum of Art.* [Master's thesis, City University of New York.] CUNY Academic Works. Retrieved on 12 May 2020 from https://academicworks.cuny.edu/cgi/viewcontent.cgi?article=1397&context=cc_etds_theses.

Smith, A. (2016). A literature review of the therapeutic mechanisms of art therapy for veterans with post-traumatic stress disorder. *International Journal of Art Therapy, 21*(2), 66–74.

Smith, M., Robinson, L. & Segal, J. (2019, October). *PTSD in Military Veterans.* HelpGuide. Retrieved on 12 May 2020 from www.helpguide.org/articles/ptsd-trauma/ptsd-in-military-veterans.htm.

Steele, E., Wood, D.S., Usadi, E. & Applegarth, D.M. (2018). TRR's Warrior Camp: An intensive treatment program for combat trauma in active military and veterans of all eras. *Military Medicine, 183*(3/4), 403–407.

Steenkamp, M.M., Litz, B.T., Gray, M.J., Lebowitz, L. *et al.* (2011). A brief exposure-based intervention for service members with PTSD. *Cognitive and Behavioral Practice, 18*, 98–107.

Stein, J.Y., Levin, Y., Aloni, R. & Solomon, Z. (2019). Psychiatric distress among aging decorated and non-decorated veterans: The role of impostorism and loneliness. *Aging & Mental Health, March,* 1–9. doi.org/10.1080/13607863.2019.1594164.

Stein, N.R., Mills, M.A., Arditte, K., Mednoza, C. *et al.* (2012). A scheme for categorizing traumatic military events. *Behavioral Modification, 36*(6), 787–807.

Sullivan, W.P. & Starnino, V.R. (2018). Moral wounds and moral repair: The dilemmas of spirituality and culturally sensitive practice. *Families in Society: The Journal of Contemporary Social Services, 110*(2), 139–150.

Suris, A., Lind, L., Kashner, M., Borman, P.D. & Petty, F. (2004). Sexual assault in women veterans: An examination of PTSD risk, health care utilization, and cost of care. *Psychosomatic Medicine, 66*, 749–756.

Suris, A., Link-Malcom, J., Chard, K., Ahn, C. & North, C. (2013). A randomized clinical trial of cognitive processing therapy for veterans with PTSD related to military sexual trauma. *Journal of Traumatic Stress, 26*, 28–37.

Thomas, J., Wilk, J., Riviere, L., McGurk, D., Castro, C. & Hoge, C. (2010). Prevalence of mental health problems and functional impairment among active component and National Guard soldiers 3 and 12 months following combat in Iraq. *Archives of General Psychiatry, 67*(6), 614–623. doi:10.1001/archgenpsychiatry.2010.54.

Thompson, G. (2009). Artistic sensibility in the studio and gallery model revisiting process and product. *Art Therapy: Journal of the American Art Therapy Association, 26*(4), 159–166. doi:10.1080/07421656.2009.10129609.

Turchik, J.A. & Wilson, S.M. (2010). Sexual assault in the U.S. military: A review of literature and recommendations for the future. *Aggression and Violent Behavior, 15*, 267–277, doi:10.1016/j.avb.2010.01.005.

U.S. Department of Defense (2012). *Department of Defense Annual Report on Sexual Assault in the Military (Volume I)*. Retrieved on 12 May 2020 from www.sapr.mil/public/docs/reports/FY12_DoD_SAPRO_Annual_Report_on_Sexual_Assault-VOLUME_ONE.pdf.

U.S. Department of Defense (2019). *Department of Defense Annual Report on Sexual Assault in the Military: Fiscal Year 2018*. Retrieved on 12 May 2020 from www.sapr.mil/sites/default/files/DoD_Annual_Report_on_Sexual_Assault_in_the_Military.pdf.

U.S. Department of Defense (2020). Annual report on sexual assault in the military: Fiscal year 2019. Retrieved on 12 May 2020 from https://media.defense.gov/2020/Apr/30/2002291660/-1/-1/1/1_DEPARTMENT_OF_DEFENSE_FISCAL_YEAR_2019_ANNUAL_REPORT_ON_SEXUAL_ASSAULT_IN_THE_MILITARY.PDF.

U.S. Department of Defense (n.d.). *History of Marine Corps Day*. Retrieved on 12 May 2020 from https://afd.defense.gov/History/Marine-Corps-Day.

U.S. Department of the Navy (2009). *OPNAVINST 5350D Navy alcohol and drug abuse prevention and control*. https://www.secnav.navy.mil/doni/Directives/05000%20General%20Management%20Security%20and%20Safety%20Services/05-300%20Manpower%20Personnel%20Support/5350.4D.pdf.

U.S. Department of Veterans Affairs (2004). *Iraq War Clinician Guide* (2nd ed.) Retrieved on 12 May 2020 from https://networkofcare.org/library/Iraq%20Clinician%20Whole%20Magilla.pdf.

U.S. Department of Veterans Affairs (2014). *Military Sexual Trauma*. https://www.mentalhealth.va.gov/docs/mst_general_factsheet.pdf .

U.S. Department of Veterans Affairs (2019a). *Military Sexual Trauma: Treatment*. Retrieved on 12 May 2020 from www.mentalhealth.va.gov/msthome/treatment.asp.

U.S. Department of Veterans Affairs (2019b). 2019 National Veteran Suicide Prevention Annual Report. Retrieved on 12 May 2020 from www.mentalhealth.va.gov/docs/data-sheets/2019/2019_National_Veteran_Suicide_Prevention_Annual_Report_508.pdf.

U.S. Government Printing Office (2006). *United States Code, 2006 Edition, Supplement 5, Title 38 – Veterans' Benefits*. Retrieved on 12 May 2020 from www.gpo.gov/fdsys/granule/USCODE-2011-title38/USCODE-2011 -title38-partII-chap17-subchapII-sec1720D.

van der Kolk, B. (2014). *The Body Keeps the Score: Brain, Mind, and Body in the Healing of Trauma*. Thousand Oaks, CA: Sage.

Vargas, A.F., Hanson, T., Kraus, D., Drescher, K. & Foy, D. (2013). Moral injury in combat veterans' narrative responses from the National Vietnam Veterans' Readjustment Study. *Traumatology, 19*(3), 243–250. doi:10.1177/1534765613476099.

Vartanian, H. (2019). *A Museum Hires a Full-Time Therapist*. Retrieved on 12 May 2020 from https://hyperallergic.com/491210/a-museum-hires-a-full-time-therapist.

Vespa, J. E. (2020). *Those who served: American's Veterans from World War II to the War on Terror.* U.S. Department of Commerce, U.S. Census Bureau. Retrieved on 12 May 2020 from www.census.gov/content/dam/Census/library/publications/2020/demo/acs-43.pdf.

Voelkel, E., Pukay-Martin, A.N.D., Walter, K.H. & Chard, K.M. (2015). Effectiveness of cognitive processing therapy for male and female U.S. veterans with and without military sexual trauma. *Journal of Traumatic Stress, 28*(3), 174–182.

Walker, M. (2015). *Melissa Walker: Unmasking the Wounds of War.* [Video file]. Retrieved on 12 May 2020 from www.tedmed.com/talks/show?id=526823.

Walker, M.S., Kaimal, G., Gonzaga, A.M.L., Myers-Coffman, K.A. & DeGraba, T.J. (2017). Active-duty military service members' visual representations of PTSD and TBI in masks. *International Journal of Qualitative Studies in Health and Well-being, 12*(1), doi:10.1080/17482631.2016.1267317.

Weil, S. (1999). From being about something to being for somebody: The ongoing transformation of the American museum. *Daedalus, 128*(3), 229–258.

Weiss, B., Azevedo, K., Webb, K., Gimeno, J. & Cloitre, M. (2018). Interpersonal regulation (STAIR) for rural women veterans who have experienced military sexual trauma. *Journal of Traumatic Stress, 31*(4), 620–625.

Wilkinson, R.A. & Chilton, G. (2013). Positive art therapy: Linking positive psychology to art therapy theory, practice, and research. *Art Therapy: Journal of the American Art Therapy Association, 30*(1), 5–11.

Wilson, C. & Moulton, B. (2010). *Loneliness Among Older Adults: A National Survey of Adults 45+.* Washington, DC

Wilson, L. (2001). Symbolism and Art Therapy. In J. Rubin (ed.), *Approaches to Art Therapy: Theory and Technique* (p.49). Philadelphia, PA: Bruner/Routledge.

Wisco, B.E., Marx, B.P., May, C.L., Martini, B. *et al.* (2017). Moral injury in U.S. combat veterans: Results from the National Health and Resilience in Veterans study. *Depression and Anxiety, 34*, 340–347.

Wix, L. (2000). Looking for what's lost: The artistic roots of art therapy: Mary Huntoon. *Art Therapy: Journal of the American Art Therapy Association, 17*(3), 168–176. doi: 10.1080/07421656.2000.10129699.

Wong, A.N.T. & Au, W.T. (2019). Effects of tactile experience during clay work creation in improving psychological well-being. *Art Therapy: Journal of the American Art Therapy Association, 36*(4), 192–199.

Yalom, Y.D. (2005). *The Theory and Practice of Group Psychotherapy.* New York, NY: Basic Books.

Yan, G.W. (2016). The invisible wound: Moral injury and its impact on the health of Operation Enduring Freedom/Operation Iraqi Freedom veterans. *Military Medicine, 181*(5), 451–458.

Zhao, L., Zhang, X. & Ran, G. (2017). Positive coping style as a mediator between older adults' self-esteem and loneliness. *Social Behavior and Personality: An International Journal, 45*(10), 1619–1628. doi.org/10.2224/sbp.6486.

Index